BEHIND EVERY CHOICE

IS A

STORY

My mother wanted to be a
loving mother but had to have
children she didn't want, more
than she had strength for. My
Dad was a minister and thought
God sent us. After five children
Mom wrote to Margaret Sanger
to find out how to prevent babies.
M.S. was in jail and could not
help. I was born and my mother
never accepted me - could not. I
never knew why until she broke
down when I was an adult and told
me. She had given up and had
three more children after me. I
have had to forgive her but it
gives me incentive to work for
the support of every child a wanted
child.

Behind Every Choice Is a Story

Gloria Feldt

with Carol Trickett Jennings

University of North Texas Press
Denton, Texas

6 5 4 3 2 1

The paper in this book meets the minimum requirements of the American
National Standard for Permanence of Paper for Printed Library Materials,
Z39.48.1984.

Permissions
University of North Texas Press
PO Box 311336
Denton, TX 76203-1336
940-565-2142

Library of Congress Cataloging-in-Publication Data
Feldt, Gloria, 1942–
Behind every choice is a story / by Gloria Feldt ; with Carol Trickett
Jennings.— 1st ed.
p.   cm.
Includes bibliographical references and index.
ISBN 1-57441-158-6 (hardcover : alk. paper)
1. Pro-choice movement—United States. 2. Birth control—
United States. 3. Abortion—United States. 4. Planned Parenthood
Federation of America—History. I. Jennings, Carol Trickett. II. Title.
HQ766.5.U5 F44 2003
363.9'6'0973—dc21
2002012608

Cover design by Patricia Adams

Dedication

For Tammy, Linda, and David who I love fiercely
and
for the women of tomorrow: their choices and their stories

I will one day leave this world for the next and I will ask my maker's forgiveness regarding many things, but preventing the birth of a child I had no way of providing for will not be one of them. . . . Who am I? I am your daughter, I am your best friend. I am your neighbor, your sister, your wife, your future mother. And I have a story . . .

—Mandy, age thirty-four

Contents

Foreword

Judging from the brouhaha occasioned by my twenty seconds of nudity on the Broadway stage in *The Graduate*, this country has an anguished relationship with its sexuality. It's fine to sell cars with sex, but to talk honestly about it, well . . . as Gloria Feldt notes in this moving and momentous book, "What are we teaching our children? That sex is dirty and awful and ugly, so save it for someone you love?"

Behind Every Choice Is a Story makes it clear that the movement for reproductive freedom holds the moral high ground despite the din of our detractors, bawling from their "bully pulpits" that teens must learn only abstinence, that contraceptives should be a controlled substance, that family planning is classified information, and that choosing abortion is wrong no matter what the circumstance.

To me, the right to make our own reproductive choices is as fundamental as the right to raise our voices in the public square. We actors are often asked to lend our familiar and forceful voices to promote causes. But I don't consider reproductive rights a "cause"—it's a calling. I am raising my voice in support of those who have dedicated their lives to that calling, so that my daughter will have the most basic freedoms as she sets forth in life to realize her dreams. It is about time, and Gloria's book inspires us to heed the clarion call, tell our stories, and raise our voices together.

There's an old saw in show business that if you want to send a message, call Western Union. Those of us who make our living on stage and screen know that engaging the hearts and minds of audiences is not about messages, it's about stories. *Behind Every Choice Is a Story* will change how America talks about reproductive rights. In my view, the pro-choice story is the truly life-enhancing story. Choice, after all, is about the whole panoply of reproductive decisions we make as we go through our lives.

How true it is that behind every reproductive choice is a story. It was true for me. I can honestly say that when I was a college student, a Planned Parenthood clinic saved—and changed—my life. I know you will identify, as I did, with many of the accounts chronicled here, and with Gloria Feldt's own life-affirming story as it threads its way through these arresting pages.

Every story in this book, no matter how uplifting or sad, in the end is a story of triumph and courage, because in a climate often hostile to reproductive freedom, just talking about sexual fulfillment or sexual abuse or sexual ignorance or life before the Pill or life before *Roe v. Wade* is an act of bravery.

But we all become stronger when we tell our stories—the individual stories that make us special and the shared stories that make us brave.

Kathleen Turner

Acknowledgments

In the course of writing *Behind Every Choice Is a Story*, I learned that a book is never finished; an author has to decide it is time to stop writing. Since I first conceptualized this book and until I finally decided it was time to stop, I have received the most amazing support and help from people who believed in me and in the importance of telling these stories. I am filled with gratitude to you all. The book could never have come to fruition without you, and it is much the richer because of your contributions.

I thank Carol Jennings whose passion for Planned Parenthood's mission made her much more than a superb writing partner. I am indebted to Marcia Ann Gillespie, Ceil Cleveland, and Cherie Carter-Scott, each of whom gave so unsparingly of their fine writers' sensibilities to read drafts and who challenged me to improve upon my work. A special thank you to Frank Rich who helped me to see that I could tell my personal story.

Many staff hands and eyes at Planned Parenthood Federation of America have touched the book, added to its content and its veracity, and shaped it with their ideas along the way. I am grateful to one and all, and especially to Patricia Adams, Alyssa Arvary, Desiree Ross Bunch and Jalen Bunch, Jim Byrnes, Helena Clarke, Shannon Criniti, Carol Dacey-Charles, Jannie Downes, Lydia Franco, Bari George, Ann Glazier, Jennifer Johnsen, Loretta Kane, Jon Knowles, Kim Lafferty, Eira Lopez and Anthony Feliciano, Jim Lubin, Colleen McCabe, Josie McGee, Vikina Mejia, Heidi Melz, Shilpa Patel, Eve Paul, Mary Philbin, Lisa Potter, Roberto Quezada, Kate Rounds, Barbara Snow, Rachel Strauber, Dawn Thomsen, Elizabeth Toledo, and Connie Watts. They are miracle workers one and all.

Proving once again that the world turns on human connections, Sharon Allison introduced me to Fran Vick who introduced me to the great folks at the University of North Texas Press. Karen DeVinney pursued me persistently and believed in the importance of this book; Ron Chrisman and Paula Oates have been so supportive and a delight to work with. I am very proud to have my first book published by a Texas press; there seems to be some kind of divine justice at work here. Nancy Land, another Texas connection, also buoyed me up by opening doors when I encountered the inevitable publishing roadblocks.

Thanks to Planned Parenthood affiliate colleagues; thanks to the people I knew, those I met along the way, and the people I will never meet, who contributed letters and stories. Each story is special. I only wish there had been room for all of them and for every word of those stories that were included. Don't worry, there will be other books.

Thanks to my daughter Linda Singh for her beautiful reminiscences of my parents and my grandmother, to my son David Bosse and my daughter Tammy Bosse for sharing their memories of our lives, and to all three of them for putting up with me for all these years. I also want to express my gratitude and love to the entire extended family too numerous to name for your interest and support. I can't give enough thanks to my husband, Alex Barbanell, who put up with my evenings and weekends of writing, shared my aspirations for the book as well as my passion for the cause of reproductive self-determination, encouraged me every step of the way, and gave my story a happy ending.

Introduction

For as long as there have been humans, there have been stories. The stories in this book chronicle what makes us human—the ability to shape our destinies. For as long as there have been humans, we have tried to determine our reproductive destinies—to have children when we want to and not to have children when we are unprepared or unable to care for them. Just as Crissy has done.

 If it weren't for you guys, a lot of people's dreams would never come true. Becoming pregnant is a scary thing. I've learned a great lesson and I never want to have to go through something like this again. I now realize that doing one little thing can ruin your entire life and mess up all your dreams. You have given me a chance to go for my dreams and succeed in life.

If I ever have [a child] I want it to have the best that I could possibly give it, with a father and mother who love it. I was an unexpected child that perhaps shouldn't have been born. But since I'm here, I'm going to strive to make things better.

You have given me the chance to live and make my life the way it should be. Thank you.

—Crissy, age sixteen

To me, this letter says it all. I have kept it since the day I received it from Crissy, years ago. I read it often. It reminds me why reproductive rights are so important. It gives me courage in the face of attacks. It inspires me to remember that behind every choice, there is a story as unique as the human being who makes it. Today, quiet, small voices like Crissy's, which express very personal and conscientious childbearing decisions, are too often drowned out by the public roar of those who would deny women the moral standing, the legal right, and the practical access to reproductive self-determination.

I have written this book because I believe we owe it to these women to let their voices ring in testimony to the fundamental human and civil right to make their own childbearing choices.

In order to retain the unique voices of the contributors, I have left the quotes from letters largely unedited. Names and other identifying factors have been changed except where the authors have kindly allowed me to identify them. Ages, where known, are actual.

Our bodies, our choices, our lives

The issues of sex and reproduction, in the reality of our individual lives, reach far beyond childbearing into every corner of our hearts, minds, and souls. To express sexual love, to nurture a family—these acts are the essence of our humanity.

I have learned from nearly three decades of my work with Planned Parenthood Federation of America (PPFA) and from my own experience as a mother that in a woman's life, these issues take on another, almost unfathomable, layer of meaning. The choices we make manifest themselves in our bodies, define our lives, and become our stories. I have also learned from reading thousands of letters and listening to so many real human stories that the issues are broad and complex: they include the relationship between reproductive choices and other life choices; the moral dilemmas that arise when worthy values compete for preeminence; and the ultimate question of who, by law or social convention, gets to make these decisions.

If you think this is a book about abortion, think again. Many stories in this book *are* about abortion, to be sure, but most are about the many other, often unacknowledged, facets of reproductive life. Here's what reproductive choice means to women, in the words of Elissa, a twenty-six-year-old mother:

 Reproductive choice gives me the opportunity to give myself totally to the kids I already have. Not having more children by choice allows me to be a bigger part of the lives of the children I have.

People often tell me they wish something as personal as childbearing decisions were not so polarized and politicized as they have become today. So do I. Telling our stories can help lead us to that place.

For when we open our hearts and listen carefully to real-life experiences, we come to understand that even the hot-button abortion issue isn't about abortion, really. Opening our hearts and minds to these experiences forces each of us to examine what we believe about the nature and purpose of human sexuality, whether women should have an equal place at life's table, how children are valued, how women's lives and bodily integrity should be respected, and how individual liberties and social justice are defined. It's about the whole person and the fullness of our lives. In short, it's about a worldview.

Yet in real life, whatever your worldview, sexual and reproductive issues beg to leave the political arena. Real human life is lived one person at a time, one choice at a time.

And behind every choice is a story

Not since Margaret Sanger, the "mother" of the birth control movement and founder of Planned Parenthood, published *Motherhood in Bondage* in 1928 have stories like these been told in this way. Like the women who wrote to her desperately seeking the knowledge that would give them control of their own lives, people today write to the organization that carries on Sanger's legacy with their heartfelt, compelling stories of despair and hope, fear and courage, defeat and triumph, ignorance and awakening.

Today's real-life stories

Today, there are many similarities with Sanger's day. The basic human concerns of sex, love, health, and wanting a better life for one's children are timeless. Yet there is a profound difference: then, women already had more children than they felt able to care for, and they wanted to know how to stop. Today, most women start using birth control before they have their first child—giving the term "family planning" full and joyous meaning.

The writers of today's stories are exceedingly diverse in age, ethnicity, geography, and more. They include men as well as women. Some write long and involved letters; others write single phrases. Letters come daily from various sources: many arrive on my desk unsolicited; some are from people who write after they've used reproductive health services; some come via the Planned Parenthood Web sites; a few are from individuals who knew I was writing this book. What they all have in common is this: each is seeking to make her or his life's dream come true.

I found that the stories grouped themselves naturally, first into personal reproductive life-cycle issues, which make up the first two sections of the book, and then into the "personally political" issues that became the last two sections. Perhaps it is not surprising that while I was assembling other people's stories, I realized my own life had followed the same pattern of personal experience, succeeded by—or perhaps triggering—political awakening, and so I decided to share my story with you, too. I became convinced that the telling of our personal stories is the most powerful antidote to political assaults.

One of the women who wrote to me is Robbie Ausley, a mother of four from Austin, Texas, who with her husband, Tom, decided to share with her college-age children, and then with her community, the story of their abortion decision. You'll read it later in the book, but here she tells us why she speaks out:

 Why have I taken the risk to share this personal experience? My story is not unique. It is the story of many women and their families who walk among us. Hopefully by putting a face on this issue, people will more fully understand the human element involved in this controversial debate and thereby be renewed with courage and compassion to continue fighting for a woman's right and need to make that decision.

Why must these stories be told right now?

Reading these stories from my vantage point as Planned Parenthood's leader today, I can see Margaret Sanger as if I am standing in a kaleidoscopic mirror with her. Our images blend with the writers of these letters. We are all reflected from a myriad of angles, just as the realities of our individual lives reflect a myriad of choices—both universal and infinitely unique.

But ominous shadows lurk in the background. They threaten to overwhelm the hopes and dreams of the people who share their stories with us. That's exactly why I feel such urgency to tell the stories now.

First, we're a long way from a world where Crissy, Elissa, Robbie, and others like them can realize their dreams. Sex is still too often treated like a dirty word in this country and sexual health is not discussed, to the detriment of our children and even adults. Many people in the U.S. and abroad lack access to the most basic reproductive health care. Our culture is only slowly learning to value girls and women as it does boys and men. And each new generation needs something different from this movement as technology and society change.

Second, the gains we have made face unprecedented challenges from those who oppose reproductive self-determination—and they are aided by a president, Congress, and state governments aligned to take our choices away. We face a political crisis of monumental proportions, a pernicious web of assaults on reproductive rights and access to reproductive health care: the global gag rule; the building of a legal platform to overturn *Roe v. Wade;* and dramatic increases in abstinence-only sex education while family planning appropriations decrease. *Roe* itself is held tenuously by a razor-thin, one-vote margin, and anti-choice President George W. Bush will almost certainly appoint the justice who will cast the deciding vote that either sustains reproductive choice or sounds its death knell.

In the thirty years since *Roe v. Wade* legalized abortion and affirmed—once and for all, we thought—a woman's right to make her own childbearing choices, the vast majority of Americans have had the luxury of taking our reproductive freedoms for granted. But in our post-September 11 world, we have all learned, tragically, that freedom's champions must be ever vigilant. And so it is with the champions of reproductive freedom.

I hope this book will serve as the clarion call, before it is too late, to save what has been won. But more importantly, my message is one of great hope and an exhortation to advance our unfinished twenty-first-century agenda. We must settle the legal right to reproductive self-determination and create a supportive social climate which includes universal access to reproductive health care services that make those rights meaningful.

I am utterly convinced that the most compelling voice of this clarion call will be our stories, not the braying of the anti-choice politician or the shrill pontifications of the talk show host. We must go back to the source—to the stories of people, like you and like me—whose lives are so profoundly affected by the freedom to choose.

My own journey is part of the story and perhaps yours is too

Today, as I stand by Margaret Sanger's side in the mirror, I see great hope and huge advances. But I also see many anguished faces among the people who write me. And I was there once. My own choices have defined my life, fueled my passion for social justice, and led me to devote my life's work to this mission. I married at fifteen and was the mother of three at twenty. My gradual awakening to the injustices that occur when women are denied fundamental human and civil rights or the services that make rights meaningful, and my concerns for the well-being of children here in the U.S. and abroad, have opened my heart even wider to the stories and choices of others. And on the most visceral level, I know I would not be here sharing these stories with you today were it not for the birth control pill that enabled me to limit my own fertility and begin to make my dreams come true.

Perhaps you, too, have a story. And if you do, I hope you will share it with me so that together we can ensure that future generations will experience the great blessings of motherhood in freedom.

Part I

Growing up

I don't think adults realize the constant pressure put on teens today. Besides the fact that you always seem to have homework, extracurricular stuff, and work, most of us 'normal' teens have these crazy little inevitable things called 'emotions.' I think most adults believe that the majority of teens just have sex and don't even think about it. But for the most of us, deciding to have sex is a big decision. Teens and adults need to take responsibility. Teens need to remember that even though it may be hard, talking to adults to get proper birth control and condoms is the safest way to ensure your health in the long run. And adults need to remember that the reason why teens feel so uncomfortable talking about these things with them is because they look down on teen sex so much that teens are scared to talk to them about it.

—Cindy, age seventeen

Chapter One
The talk

When the question is sex, the answer is silence.

My mother visited me in New York City a few years ago. One day, as we were walking home from Rockefeller Center, she said to me, out of the blue, "You know, I don't think I ever said the word 'sex' to you in my life." I thought for a minute. Because of my job, I probably spend more time talking about sex than any woman in America.

"You know," I said. "I think you're right." As best I can recall, that constitutes the sum total of our discussions of the subject. So I could feel for Tamika:

 My mother was not at ease talking about sex or even about the female body. I was at Girl Scout Camp when I woke up to a sleeping bag full of blood and thought I was dying. I was too afraid to even talk to our troop leaders. A week later my mother discovered, from looking at the laundry, what was going on. She never talked to me about exactly what happened but she did provide a pamphlet . . . I just thank God that I did *not* end up a statistic—a pregnant teen.

—Tamika, age twenty-eight

America's most popular topic is its most avoided subject

When I was thirteen, my father handed me a slim paperback titled *The Facts of Life and Love for Teenagers.* Not that he ever said anything else to me, but at least I had some accurate biological information and, in a larger sense, acknowledgment that I was growing up and therefore entitled to know these things. He probably felt pleased to have fulfilled his duty as a parent. My little book became the hottest item at that summer's Campfire Camp. By the end of my two-week stay, the book was in shreds. Like most children, my campmates learned about sex from a peer—me (or at least my book). And my career as a sexuality educator was unwittingly launched. The only problem—other than the fact that my little book was trashed—was that I didn't understand much of what I had read, and I was too embarrassed to ask questions. No one in my home said "sex."

Ancient history? I wish. Not enough has changed. From Jeni, now nineteen and in college:

> The frustration, the pain, the shame and guilt. I was only fifteen and I didn't know what else to do. My little sister was pregnant also. We both had just recently lost our virginities and I still didn't even know what an orgasm was. In my house we talked about everything, but that one topic seemed to stay out of all conversation.

Jeremy, twenty-one, says it even more succinctly:

> As a teenager, I was not informed of sex . . . by my parents or schools. I had to learn it all on my own, the hard way.

In public today, battle lines about sex are drawn all the time. Over condoms. Over sex education. Over what services a teen courageous enough to go to a family planning clinic can get. Comprehensive, medically accurate sex education gets painted as promoting sex and promiscuity. Contraceptive ads are banished from Fox TV 's sexually explicit *Temptation Island*. At the same time, in private, parents retreat from honest talk about sex. Doctors fail to take sexual histories. School nurses cower. Talk is perceived as risky. A parent who merely teaches a child proper terminology for body parts can get into trouble, as Marian found out when her daughter was in daycare:

 The little boy said, do you want to see my peter? My daughter replied, "that's not called a peter, it is a penis!!" I was called in by the school principal because the boy went home and told his mother that my daughter told him he had a penis. Later, my daughter was in the girl's bathroom while a teacher was changing her 'pad'. My daughter went out to a class of five-year-olds and announced that the teacher's egg broke. Needless to say, I was called to the principal's office again. This time they recommended that I tell my daughter that not everyone is ready for the information she has. Somehow, she is a well-adjusted twenty-five-year-old going to college full time and working full time. She has decided to go the route of abstinence.

There is more to Marian's story. Sexually abused as a child, promiscuous as a teen ("looking for love in all the wrong places," as she puts it), at eighteen she gave birth to a daughter whom she surrendered for adoption. Soon she had two more daughters but divorced the father and raised them alone. She believes many of her problems arose because she had been uninformed about sex when she was growing up, and so she made sure her own children's questions were answered honestly.

Conflicts such as Marian encountered continue because, paradoxically, sex is both America's most popular topic and its most avoided subject. We have sexual schizophrenia. Sex is sold every day as cosmetics and cars. Yet it took an act of political courage for the U.S. Surgeon General, Dr. David Satcher, to tell the truth about sex and sexual health in America when he issued his *Call to Action to Promote Sexual Health and Responsible Sexual Behavior* in mid-2001.

Breaking the silence about sex

It's hard to talk to your kids about sex. They ask embarrassing questions. They ask you the questions before you are ready with the answers, and they need to know *now*. They'll take you places you don't want to go, areas of your own life that are uncomfortable or involve difficult memories. What do their questions mean? Are they actually having sex or just curious? You may want them to wait until marriage or at least until they are older, but did you? And at some point you'll have to acknowledge that your children are sexual beings. This is not easy, but think of the consequences when we don't. Melinda and her parents, too, learned the hard way:

 I am sixteen years old and I already have a baby. If I would have known about birth control ten months ago I would have been able to prevent this unexpected pregnancy. Like many other young girls, I didn't have advice from my parents about contraceptives; face it parents are not comfortable with their teens sexuality.

Another sixteen-year old, Janelle, is a budding sex educator trying to help her peers:

 Recently, I was having a conversation with several girls from my high school. They were asking me specific questions about my choice to get the Depo-Provera shot and prevent myself from pregnancy. I was shocked at the questions they were asking me, and I realized that they were very uncertain and uninformed about what they could be and should be doing to keep themselves healthy and to prevent pregnancy while they were sexually active. Most of them did not fully understand the purpose or procedure of a Pap smear, and didn't understand why they should have one once they became sexually active. Many of the girls were primarily worried about telling their parents about their decisions . . . the school responds by simply turning their heads at the sight of the ever increasing numbers of pregnant girls in the hallways. I am trying to take action against this policy of ignoring the sexual uncertainty at my school, and I am looking for help.

This mom from Iowa thought she had the tools to make things different for her daughters than they were for her—until she realized it wasn't just about biology:

 I considered myself a modern mom, comfortable with everything, including human sexuality. That plus my scientific approach made me confident that discussions about sex would be frank and open, and I'd be objective on all aspects of their developing sexuality. Early in my veterinary career, much of my work focused on reproductive physiology. Dinner table discussions often included descriptions of collecting semen from stallions, artificial insemination, and pelvic exams of mares and cows. The kids saw mares being bred, and once saw a calf being born. The girls asked lots of questions, and I answered them thoroughly, often with the help of anatomy books. They quickly extrapolated the mechanics of animal reproduction to human reproduction, at which time I pulled out my human anatomy book and completed the picture for them. I was sure I had laid the perfect framework for their journey through adolescence.

When my oldest daughter was fifteen, I walked in on her and her boyfriend on the floor kissing. They jumped up. I could see the boyfriend had an erection the size of Texas, and my daughter's bra appeared to be askew. I went through an astonishing range of emotions: horror, incredulity, fear, anger, guilt, and finally, amazement. I was amazed that I had been naive enough to think I could manage my child's sexual development with clinical objectivity. I was completely unable to deal with the reality that she would actually *have sex.* I immediately made an appointment at the Women's Health Clinic and briefed the physician's assistant about my concerns and my inability to cope. What I gave my daughter at fifteen was unquestioned access to high-quality, confidential health care—from someone who was better than I was at the job, in spite of all my "objectivity." Today, my daughter is a healthy, twenty-one-year-old college student.

What parent hasn't had such a "wake-up" moment? The first time my daughter found a tampon and asked me what it was, I hyperventilated. I was tongue-tied—I'd promised myself I'd do better than my mother but had not a clue how to do that. All I could do at first was to bumble around, scared to death to talk and scared to death not to talk. It's not like anyone has any unique body parts or functions. It's just that I had no role models to fall back on as I began to try to break the silence about sex. I wasn't very successful, as my children have since told me.

The cost of silence is immense. Children are learning about sex. But when parents don't talk and schools don't teach, they get most of their information from media hype or from their peers—friends and young relatives—and a good bit of that information is inaccurate or misleading or incomplete.

 I was sixteen years old and was involved in a relationship with a nineteen-year-old guy from my neighborhood. We were not using any kind of protection (which was available to me at anytime, but we were both too embarrassed to buy it), but I thought that I could figure out when I was ovulating by avoiding having sex after my period. Well, I figured wrong. I was sixteen, in high school and pregnant. My family would not approve of this so I could not tell them.

—Sarah, age eighteen

Looking for a safe place in cyberspace

Increasingly, teens are looking for information on the Internet, and although there are reliable Web sites, getting to them can mean wading through a slough of pornography and even sexual predators. The teens who bring their questions to teenwire®.com, a Planned Parenthood Web site for teens, are concerned about their changing bodies, about what's normal, about whether they are ready to have sex. Some ask how to talk to their parents about sex.

These examples of questions asked of teenwire.com demonstrate the uncomfortable combination of ignorance and sophistication that characterizes today's teenagers:

❋ I think I am pregnant what should I do I can't tell my mom . . . so what should I do I don't wanna go to the hospital so what should I do?

❋ I am almost sixteen years old and I have not started my period. Sometimes I touch myself down "there" and I am wondering if that will prevent my period?

❋ We always use condoms every time we have sex—except the last time. Could I be pregnant?

❋ You can't get pregnant from oral sex, can you?

I don't envy today's parents. There is a frequently run Partnership for a Drug-Free America ad that shows a boy with his hand over his mouth and an embarrassed look on his face. The caption says, "It's not half as uncomfortable as talking to your kids about sex." How poignant that so many parents find this to be true. Many studies have found that parents and teens have very different perspectives about whether they have talked about sex and what they have talked about when they did talk about it. For example, 72 percent of mothers say they have talked with their teens about sex, but only 45 percent of their teens agree. Similarly, only one-third of teens say they've had "a good talk" about sex with their fathers.

Two sixteen-year-olds report their experiences below. The two stories turned out differently because the first had access to a trustworthy source of information and health services and the second did not:

 I am a sixteen-year-old girl. I've been sexually active for the past six months. My boyfriend and I love each other very much and we knew we were ready for sex. The only thing that was holding me back for a while was the fear of getting an STI [sexually transmitted infection] or becoming pregnant. I know a lot of people say to talk to your mom, she's been there and all that, but realistically, not everyone's mom is willing to discuss that, much less know her baby girl is having sex. And my mom is one of those people. Without access to contraceptives, I might be another teenage statistic.

 This was the very first time I had ever been in any kind of women's health center [pregnancy]. My mother never wanted me to get a Pap test, so this was my first experience in the stirrups. I was *very* scared.

What's so unfortunate about this disconnect is that teens who perceive they have a better level of communication with their parents are less likely to engage in sexual intercourse. But I know from my own life that translating a study like this into real life is not easy. If measured against my parents and the time into which I was born, I was more open with my children about sex. But I realized too late that the culture had changed so much that "better" wasn't good enough to meet the needs of kids coming of age in the '70s. My children were exposed to so much more than I was—incredible social upheaval, all-pervasive mass media, and, of course, the sexual revolution. I didn't fully understand the needs and pressures of their lives in their era. I suppose this happens in every generation. But it haunts me because I wanted it to be different for them.

Today's kids—and their parents—face even more. Mass media makes sexually explicit materials available twenty-four/seven with very little responsible context. In the past twenty years, HIV/AIDS has raised the stakes of "the talk" to matters of life and death. Parents are rightly afraid, and this fear alone may be propelling more parents to talk to their children—at least about this particular public health issue and its dangers. And many schools have HIV/AIDS education even if they have no other sex education. Yet an understanding of the joy of sexual love is missing when conversations about sex are couched only in terms of disease, fear, danger, and life-threatening outcomes. It's no surprise, then, that few of us grow up knowing that sexuality is a healthy, normal part of human life that greatly enriches our lives, when managed responsibly. And I weep for the millions of children who grow up without honest, real communication about sexuality. I weep for the millions of adults for whom, as a result, sex becomes identified with shame, guilt, and embarrassment instead of healthy, loving relationships.

When I read *The Facts of Life and Love for Teenagers,* I at least got the basic anatomical facts. What I didn't grasp were the emotions, the relationship issues, and the complicated interplay between the physical and emotional aspects of sex. You don't get that out of a book. You get it from years of honest, ongoing dialogue at home, in the classroom, at church or synagogue or mosque, in youth organizations. You get it from good role models of healthy relationships, sound values, and healthy sexuality, from parents who step up to their responsibilities as primary sex educators for their children in word and deed. Being told "just say no" doesn't help because "no" is not a value or a goal. And what ultimately matters in life, after all, is what we say "yes" to.

When parents, schools, and other social institutions don't help our teens get the answers they need, the result is the high rate of unintended pregnancy, abortion, and sexually transmitted infections that plague the United States. The personal and social costs of our silence stand in stark contrast to the more positive indicators of sexual health in similar countries with more open attitudes toward sex—countries like Canada, France, Great Britain, the Netherlands, and Sweden that have comprehensive, medically accurate, real sex education, easy access to contraception, and social attitudes that support sexual health.

 Wouldn't the world be a wonderful place if all daughters could talk to their parents about being sexually active?

—Jessica, age seventeen

The abstinence-only movement— abstinence of common sense

I have a feeling that most parents—including the parents of all the young women whose stories appear here, including the many parents who themselves had premarital sex—have managed to convey one message about sex: "Don't do it." (You have to figure out what "it" is yourself.) Abstinence-only sex education is not only *not* new. It always has been and is now the dominant form of sex education in America. That's the problem. And the jury is not out—every indicator of sexual health shows it does not work. It's like another drug education commercial—the one that says "Just Say No." There is a key difference. We never want our children to use drugs, but we do want them to eventually have healthy sex lives and we want them to be safe when they do have sex—even if they have sex before we think they should. So what are we teaching them instead? Sex is dirty and awful and ugly, so save it for someone you love?

Look at the trends and you can see how ignorance is expanding. Over a five-year period ending in 2002, approximately $500 million in federal and state matching funds have been spent on abstinence-only education within the welfare reform program alone. Increases in federal abstinence-only funds are coming so fast, it's hard to keep track, but annually, they are now well over $100 million. President George W. Bush's budgets have proposed huge escalations each year, despite the fact that these programs are of unproven effectiveness and potentially even harmful. I know that the abstinence-only-and-don't-ask-questions message was strong in my West Texas home, just a few miles down the road from where George W. Bush also grew up in the 1950s. It didn't work then either.

To think that these messages are the only kind being given in so many of our schools today is beyond belief but all too true—and government-enforced to boot. Sexuality is the only subject about which we would ever tolerate the notion that our young people shouldn't be well-educated and prepared for life's responsibilities ahead. It's abstinence—oops, absence—of common sense. And it is dangerous. These young people's stories give voice to the problem:

 I think I might have hiv because I gave oral sex to my boyfriend and after I had to pee a lot and then it burned and also blood came out. I told my mom about it but it went a way after I told her—what does all of this mean?

—Nikki, age seventeen

 When I was young neither of my parents talked to me about sex, so I 'learned' from friends. I was taught that if the boy 'pulls out' before ejaculation that you can't get pregnant. Surprise! I was nineteen, in college and pregnant.

—Joni, age twenty-two

I have three sisters ranging from ages twenty to twenty-four. They all had children before they were eighteen, two of them were only sixteen at the time. I am the youngest girl and I just turned eighteen. I am about to graduate from high school and attend college in August. With the education about sex I have received from my sisters, I am able to be a better person and make better decisions.

—April, age eighteen

What parents want is not what parents get

A staggering majority of parents—over 80 percent—want the schools to teach comprehensive, medically accurate sex education, including human growth and development, decision-making skills, abstinence, contraception, and prevention of sexually transmitted infections. The biggest problem is that parents generally think schools are doing the job. They think this because it belies common sense to think otherwise. Yet the number of secondary educators who say they discuss abstinence and only abstinence in their classes has increased elevenfold since 1988, from 2 percent to 23 percent. Fewer than 5 percent of students receive comprehensive sex education, and fewer still each year because of the abstinence movement. That's irresponsible and potentially dangerous. Students in comprehensive sex education classes do not have sex more often or earlier than others, but they do use contraception and practice safer sex more consistently when they become sexually active. A study in the Archives of Pediatric and Adolescent Medicine underscores the importance of starting early: teaching children about sex before they begin to make sexual choices positively influences the choices they eventually make.

Like most parents, Elvia knows that she can use all the help she can get as she balances the science of reproduction and disease with the emotionally charged issues of relationships, feelings, values, how to say "no" to sex, and what saying "yes" might mean:

I have just shown my son highlights from this month's teenwire.com newsletter. I just had to write and commend and thank you for helping me out. Although I talk with Mark a lot, and we have good communication, your newsletter supplements and complements what I try and teach him. I believe there could be a lot more understanding and communication between all of us and our children if we would allow them to become exposed to things like this that are really just part of life.

By not engaging our children in that dialogue at every opportunity, we abdicate to their peers and to the media our responsibility for teaching our children not just what sex educators fondly refer to as "the plumbing" but our personal values as well. Because talking to our kids about sex doesn't mean relinquishing our values and personal beliefs—it means giving children the tools to live them in their daily lives. By not insisting on comprehensive sexuality education in the schools, we squander the opportunity to ensure that our children understand our broader shared values too, such as respect for others and honest communication, and to teach them how to apply these values in sexual decision-making and peer pressure situations.

Real talk: many parents are doing more of it

We can do much better and I think the time is right to do just that. We can talk honestly with our children and with each other. We can hold the media accountable, and we can fight for real talk: medically accurate, comprehensive sex education in our schools, at school board meetings, and in the halls of Congress. We can take control of the public debate so it focuses on productive policies rather than extreme positions.

As I travel around the country, I see very positive trends on the personal level all the time: more parents today want to do a better job of educating their children about sexuality than our parents did for us. Their stories warm my heart and give me hope. They deserve to be supported in every way by the rest of us:

I had a child nearly seventeen years ago. I was a senior in high school. I came from a family where teen pregnancy was not necessarily accepted, but expected! Why? Because birth control was not discussed as an option. When I think about the hardships I faced as a teen mother, and the less-than-ideal circumstances my child was brought into, I get angry that my parents didn't think of me, or their potential unborn grandchildren enough to discuss birth control. My daughter, now almost seventeen, is very educated about her options, her sexual health and responsibility.

—Anna, age thirty-three

 When I found out my daughter was on birth control pills without my prior knowledge I was a bit worried. But I brought her to the clinic and we both talked to the counselor. While I'm still not overly enthused over her being sexually active, I am relieved that she's being responsible.

—James, age forty-four

Elena's story starts with a shotgun marriage at fourteen, after she left her high school campus and ended up spending the night with her boyfriend "not knowing it would change my life forever," as she put it. She had her first son at fifteen, then two more in rapid succession. She didn't know much about birth control. The stresses of finances, lack of child care and transportation, and inadequate housing contributed to a rocky marriage and a feeling of being overwhelmed. So when her own sons became teens, her concerns for them were strong. She vowed to break the cycle:

 We started discussing sex and STD's around the dinner table and just in general. The boys had a lot of questions, and I gave them the answers. On the one hand, they had information brought to them, verbally, and more pamphlets they could ask for. On the other hand, they were not given the option of having sex at a young age (under eighteen, wishful thinking), much less unprotected sex. We freely discussed condoms and abstinence. My oldest son started having sex at the age of sixteen, my second son at age seventeen, and my youngest at eighteen. To this day, condoms are still being used; the talks about safe sex, abstinence, and other methods of birth control continue.

Nine months ago, my granddaughter was born. Her father is twenty-seven and she was a planned child. I consider this to be a success story simply because the cycle of having children at an early age was broken. I feel that all the information I passed on to my sons led them to delay sex and fatherhood.

Sometimes a caring teacher, like Kathy whose story follows, bucks the system and provides help too:

 When I was teaching high school, I made it a point to spend thirty minutes every day stressing the importance of "don't make babies!" I had to do this not only because I lost several bright teenage girls to pregnancy, but to make matters worse, the extreme pro-lifers would periodically storm the campus in the morning, before school started. They distributed dead-baby cartoons as well as "messages from Jesus" insisting that he would no longer love you and would send you straight to hell for killing your baby! They not only disrupted an entire day of learning, but failed to offer contraception or even abstinence as a possible solution. Oddly enough, people who tend to be pro-life tend to be anti-welfare—who's going to raise those babies? Birth control needs to be taught, even encouraged, in schools, if we want our children to have the best future possible. The economically disadvantaged kids have too much to deal with already — proper family planning could level the playing field.

Now that I am a grandmother, I have the pleasure of watching my children improve upon my attempts at sex education. Recently, though, I was reminded that most children still learn from their peers. My husband, Alex, and I picked up three-year-old Eli and five-year-old Millan from school one day. The three "boys" were arguing jovially about who was in charge of the car. (I was driving, but never mind.) Alex thought he was playing the trump card when he said, "I am the king and your grandmother is the queen."

Little Eli, his raised hand punctuating the important facts he was imparting, declared, "Yes! And the king has a penis and the queen has labia!" "You are right, Eli," I said, after I retrieved my chin from the floor. "Where did you learn that?" I had given my daughter Linda a wonderful new book by leading sex educator Robie Harris and assumed that was the source of his great epiphany. "From Ajanta," he replied, referring to his six-year-old playmate.

Well, at least they are calling the body parts by their proper names these days, I thought, even though they are still learning from their peers. That's progress. But you'll note that my chin still hit the floor. Yes, Mother, I thought, hard as it is, even for me, we have to take a deep breath and say the word "sex" early, often, publicly, privately, and without embarrassment.

Real sex education: what the doctor ordered

Dr. David Satcher, the former surgeon general of the U.S., issued his *Call to Action* in June 2001: "Based on the scientific evidence, we face a serious public health challenge regarding the sexual health of our nation. Doing nothing is unacceptable. More than anyone, it is our children who will suffer the consequences of our failure to meet these responsibilities."

Dr. Satcher's report said:

> ➤ 87 percent of the cases of the ten most common infectious diseases are sexually transmitted diseases.

➤ An estimated 104,000 children are sexually abused each year.

➤ One-fifth of all young (ten to seventeen) Internet users have received unwanted sexual solicitations.

➤ More than one-half of all television programming has sexual content, yet responsible sexual behavior is rarely depicted.

His report calls for an honest, mature, national dialogue on sexual health, public policy informed by science and respectful of diversity, and sex education that is thorough, wide-ranging, begins early, and continues into adulthood. Sex education in school is necessary, he said, because families differ in their knowledge level about sex and human development, and in how comfortable they are discussing such things with their children.

Dr. Satcher called for:

➤ A national dialogue on responsible sexuality.

➤ Culturally and age-appropriate sex education offered at every available venue—the home, schools, churches, the media.

➤ Targeting the most vulnerable members of society—the economically disadvantaged, racial and ethnic minorities, persons with different sexual identities, disabled persons, and adolescents.

➤ Ensuring that everyone has access to sexual health and reproductive health care.

➤ Preventing sexual abuse and coercion.

Chapter Two

Strong girl, jelly woman

 I'm afraid if I don't let him do what he wants, he will leave me.
Then I feel like I have nobody, not even myself.

—Lilly, age fourteen

The loss of the self

I can close my eyes today, forty-five years later, and feel that wobbly feeling in my gut that signaled the strength to stand my ground, to hold onto my very self, was melting away—melting into jelly. I was fifteen and thought I was in love. I was smart, I came from a "good" family, and I could set goals about many other things and reach them. But I definitely didn't know how to set boundaries in relationships or feel like I could or should.

Girls face a triple whammy on the path to womanhood. It starts with lack of knowledge—lack of factual knowledge and lack of the self-knowledge that follows from not knowing the facts. Then there is the shame about sexuality that comes from our society's silence about it. Shame and the lack of knowledge are bound together by cultural cues about gender roles into a toxic combination that turns many a strong girl—a confident, adventurous, preadolescent girl (think Pippi Longstocking)—into a teenage jelly woman who molds her personality and her body to fit what she thinks the world around her, but most especially the world of teenage boys, wants her to be. Carol Gilligan, in her 1993 book, *In a Different Voice,* chronicled the change that girls go through after about age eleven—the shift from confident preteen to insecure teenager who trades sports and books for boys and beauty tips.

The loss of self permeates the letters I receive. It is so pervasive in the stories of teenage anguish that sometimes I think, "Didn't I just read that one? It must be a duplicate." I rifle through the file, and lo and behold, it isn't the same one after all. The stories are so similar that they could have been written by the same person. They start with, "I found myself pregnant," or "I went along," or "I was afraid he would leave me." Many stories tell of sexual abuse stemming from sexual ignorance and disparities in power and age. The stories have another common thread: "My parents wouldn't talk about sex and birth control."

Only rarely do girls write about being told that they have the power to say no and to say yes to each of life's choices, and it is their perfect right to make their choices for their own reasons, not for the pleasure or purposes of others. Young people will, after all, be in situations where they will have sexual feelings and they will have to deal with them, whether or not we have helped them acquire the knowledge, the skills, and the ego strength to make choices in a positive, self-affirming way.

The jelly and the mold

It's not just about hormones, though we ignore that explosive ingredient at our peril. It's a lot about the cultural mold that shapes the "jelly" of an emerging self. And how we define the nature and purpose of human sexuality and the role of women helps to shape the mold. But dig a little deeper, and all of these factors are really about who holds the culturally sanctioned power and how badly they want to keep it. That's why even today, so many young women—25 percent of those between the ages of fifteen and twenty-four, in one study—say that although they had consented to their first experience of sexual intercourse, they hadn't entirely wanted it to happen. They are often ambivalent. They wanted to, but they didn't want to at the same time.

Even when early sexual activity is fully consensual, as we must acknowledge it most often is, the prevailing "just say no" philosophy of sex education leaves teens in real-life situations where it is impossible to say "no" with strength and conviction because they don't know what saying "yes" would mean to their bodies or their lives. The ability to make considered and responsible decisions to have sex or not requires first an ability to claim the right to one's own sexuality and second the knowledge of the facts and consequences. Absent that power, the result is predictable—and heartbreaking.

 The first time I had sex I was only fourteen, and I was definitely not ready. I was in a relationship for all the wrong reasons (low self-esteem, wanted to be popular, etc.) and then I knew that the guy had a reputation for being a little pushy when it came to sex.

When it actually came down to the point where we were both half naked, tons of questions kept popping into my head. Am I really ready for this? Why am I letting it go this far? What does this mean to me? Why am I not stopping him? I ignored all of my doubts, and that horrible feeling in my gut, and went along with it.

—Jennifer, age seventeen

 Being the new girl in an extremely small school . . . I was immediately ostracized by the majority of females and quickly became the center of attention for the males. Out of a desperate need to fit in, I became associated with the wrong group of kids. One of which had an older brother who paid lots of attention to me. He flattered my damaged ego and provided me with a much-needed ally. He turned me against my family and there began a year of mental, physical, and sexual abuse.

—Samantha, age seventeen

 I never felt secure and I was always waiting for the phone to ring or for them to come over—never on time, sometimes not at all. I became very depressed.

—Julia, age seventeen

There are only two options to break this mold—hide children in a closet or teach them forthrightly what they need to know. Girls ought to be required to get a black belt in emotional self-defense.

The myth of sexual innocence

In *An End to Shame,* sociologist Ira Reiss says, "Our children will be sexual whether we participate in helping them learn about sex or not. We can neglect our responsibility to sexually educate our young children. We can make them naïve; we can make them vulnerable to abuse; we can set them up for many future sexual problems; but no matter how hard we try, we cannot make them 'sexually innocent.'"

I had a serious case of *déjà vu* all over again when this letter came across my desk from a woman twenty-five years my junior:

 I was fifteen years old when I became pregnant by the 'love of my life'. I knew it would last forever. Thank God my mother knew better. She worked for Planned Parenthood in Odessa, Texas. I really thought I wanted to be a parent. I was the only child of divorced parents, and I knew the baby would make me happy. I ended up having an abortion in a doctor's office in Odessa and my Mom was there to hold my hand afterwards. She even bought me coloring books, which is what I should have been doing instead of having sex in the first place. I have never had any regrets. I am now a thirty-four-year-old mother of a fourteen-year-old and nine-year-old triplets, identical at that. I love my four daughters and wouldn't trade them for anything in the world, but I am so thankful that I did not become a parent at fifteen! I ended up marrying the man who got me pregnant at fifteen, and after I gave birth at nineteen (way too young) we divorced. I have now been happily married for eleven years, and I have already told my oldest daughter that teen pregnancy won't take place in this house. She knows too many girls already who have basically ruined their lives thinking they would have a happy family at fifteen. Wake up, America! Talk to your children, let them know that teens having babies is not acceptable behavior!

—Wendy, age thirty-three

That I started my career with Planned Parenthood in the Odessa, Texas, oil patch in 1974 is, of course, relevant. That I first arrived in Odessa as a pregnant fifteen-year-old who really thought she wanted to be the wife of her high school sweetheart and a parent at that tender age, believing it would last forever, is also relevant. That this young woman and I could both attribute some of our angst to our dysfunctional families (real or perceived) is fairly typical for teens. That we both reached the same conclusion about the need to talk to our children and tell them that teens having babies is not acceptable, and that we are both pro-choice as a result of our personal stories—well, that's a slam dunk, even though we chose different options.

Molding jelly woman: role models and twenty kinds of toast

How does a fifteen-year-old get the kind of ideas about love and relationships and life that the Odessa letter writer and I seemed to have had?

Where does jelly woman come from?

She comes from that point in adolescence when girls realize only boys are rewarded for being strong and mature. The point where boys are expected to turn into slobs, and girls are encouraged to use the newest makeup. From "boys will be boys" and girls will be virgins. From all the negative messages girls receive about their value to and their role in society: yes, *still receive*—we haven't come nearly far enough, baby.

She comes from living with conflicted role models like my most important one, my very smart, strong grandmother, who always deferred to the men in her life. She had been a well-educated professional woman, a mathematics teacher and schoolmistress in Russia before she came to this country to marry my grandfather. This was not lost on my young consciousness. She had given it all up to move to a new country and marry a man she hadn't seen in seven years. This was not lost on me either.

After her husband died and left her with two preadolescent children, she was faced with running the family business. There is little doubt in my mind that Grandmother could have run General Motors if she had so chosen. But she always made sure a man was in charge. She made her aspirations for me clear from my earliest years—I should get a good education (just in case I needed something to fall back on) and a good husband.

The latter goal must have been foremost on my mind when my parents moved us to Stamford, Texas, a small red-dirt cotton farming community in West Texas. The town was defined by football and rodeo, rather than football and the movie theater, but otherwise, I lived in *The Last Picture Show*. Author Ceil Cleveland, who really did come from Archer City, Texas, the town depicted in *The Last Picture Show*, gives this absolutely accurate description: "[T]he boys' world—the legitimate world—of football, rodeos, learning to cuss, and dreaming about girls, was the world of Texas in that era. Girls had bit parts. We could play if we learned our lines and attempted no ad lib."

I was thirteen at the time of the move, a teenager going into ninth grade, and I decided that since I was having my life ruined by moving to a new place, I would make the best of it by remolding myself into a popular, all-American girl. I'd had a nice circle of girlfriends in Temple, Texas, before we moved, and we did many interesting things, from bicycling all over town to publishing a neighborhood newsletter, but we weren't the "in" kids. I found my peers in Stamford to be much more aggressive in talking about sex (as though they knew what they were talking about—their hunger for my sex education book makes their lack of real knowledge clear). In particular, the boys were quite aggressive in making observations about physical appearance, especially sexual attractiveness. I was unprepared, ignorant about much of what they were talking about, and I wanted to be accepted in my new hometown.

I set out to be known as sociable, friendly, and well liked instead of an achiever. I still got good grades (in my family, you either got an A, or were considered to be failing), but my classes were not difficult, so I could easily coast. I took home economics with the other girls and learned to make twenty kinds of toast. If a girl was intelligent and able, she could be a social misfit. Or she could hide her light under a bushel basket and be socially accepted. Easy choice.

I was elected sophomore class favorite and then junior class vice president. In the beginning of my junior year, while I was in Dallas with my family, I was elected cheerleader unanimously without even trying out. Mission accomplished. I had overcome not only the burden of my own intelligence, but that other teenage horror— differentness. We were new, and the only Jewish family in town. My father's western wear manufacturing plant was one of the few major businesses in town, and my mother, unlike most mothers of the time, worked with him. I knew I was too different for comfort when I received a letter from a friend addressed only "To the Eldest Daughter of Big Max, Stamford, Texas."

A girl's relationship with her father makes a big difference in her self-awareness and sense of mastery—the raw material that can help her create her own mold. When I was three, my larger-than-life father bought me the most wonderful electric train and did not find it odd that I preferred it to playing with dolls. Like many men who come from meager backgrounds, he relished buying grown-up toys for himself, when he began making enough money to do so. He took me flying in his Beechcraft Bonanza just for fun. He included me in conversations with other adults and on trips with my mother. He wanted me to have advantages he didn't have growing up in a poor immigrant family. He wanted me to go to boarding school in Dallas and college in the East—how different is that?

My mother, Florence, was extremely intelligent and capable like her own mother—and exceeded her own mother in her deference to my father. For a myriad of reasons—most of which are understandable, given her history as an insecure child who missed her father very much and never felt appreciated by her mother—my mother was an unhappy woman as long as I can remember. Her bitterness sapped my energy and could reduce me to unexpected tears in an instant. It was a huge, heavy, gray, gloomy cloud smothering the tendrils of my developing self as they searched for the nurturing sun. She could suck the sunshine out of a day with her withering assessments of the thunderstorm that would inevitably ruin it all.

My grandmother would compliment me by saying, "Gloria's so quiet, you never know you have a child around," while my father would say, "You can do anything your pretty little head desires." My mother was as passive as my father was aggressive—they had perfectly complementary neuroses. Those contradictory role models struggled for dominance within me.

About the time my hormones started running amok and my strong girl had taken those cultural clues and hidden behind the cheerleader's megaphone, my father's business started foundering and the situation at home worsened. Jelly woman opted out of this chaotic picture. I was not strong enough to stand and fight for my own identity. Instead, I melted into a new identity mold. My picture of my ideal future was far simpler: packing my husband's lunch, living a very organized life in a cute little house that I cleaned myself, with a cute baby, looking very cute myself in clothes I had made just like my friends' mothers did.

And so in that summer of 1957, I got what I had always wanted—to be "normal": the average all-American girl. Little did I know that the most average part of it was that the country registered its highest teen pregnancy data the year that I became a part of that statistic. Increasingly—not willfully though I could be quite willful in other situations—I became enchanted with the idea of being in love and living happily ever after in domestic bliss. I had a boyfriend who was in love with me and that was magnetic. Like so many of the young women whose stories come to me today, it didn't feel like a decision to have sex, though of course it was.

Not to decide is to decide. I know that now. But to the jelly woman me then, it felt as if gradually, inevitably, I was being drawn into a gently undulating tide pool from which I could never again extricate myself. I was engaged in a grown-up charade that became real life.

That fall, just after I had sewn my blue corduroy cheerleader skirt, my nineteen-year-old boyfriend and I announced to my parents that I was married, pregnant, and moving to Odessa. The silence around sex had come to its inevitable, crashing, conclusion. To save face for everyone, I felt I had to swallow my own fear and shame and tell my family I was married rather than to admit that I was just another frightened, pregnant fifteen-year-old and desperately needed their help. And all hell broke lose, as well it should have.

The paradoxical need for roots and wings

The journey through adolescence to adulthood can be difficult and painful for both boys and girls. Contrary to what we, as parents, seem to want to believe, the high school years are not always a carefree culmination of idyllic childhood. The paradox of the teen years is that teens need both roots and wings. The things that make adults crazy—risk-taking behavior, all kinds of experimentation, questioning authority, rebellion—can place teens in harm's way but also are absolutely necessary to their development as independent adults. They desperately need the roots of our values and boundaries. Yet we sabotage our ability to help steer young people through the storm and provide safe harbor when our approach is too moralistic or inflexible.

 I want to talk to a psychiatrist because there are just some things I can't tell my parents but I want adult help from somewhere. My parents wanted to know why I couldn't just talk to them. Well I did talk to them and I told them I was gay and that I had a girlfriend and now my dad thinks it's a big joke and he laughs about it all the time . . . it hurts.

—Sandy, age sixteen

 I am on this endless path
to finding who I am, what I am,
who or what I can be, in life
if I let my feelings go to my
so-called "friends" of mine
would they shy away?
I bet they'd give me the silent treatment
that can kill a person
from the inside out
so I guess I'll just sit here
in doubt
I guess I'm just scared of me

—Colleen, age fifteen

And parents are scared too, of saying too little or too much, or sending the wrong messages. How can parents trust that the lessons of the early years will eventually prevail, and their children will emerge intact on the other side of adolescence? How can they remain involved in their children's lives in ways that will help teens through these rocky times? Goodness knows, as a mother I made my share of mistakes, foremost among them, communicating too little, from which I offer some observations that may be of use to others:

Four reality checks

First, here's a reality check. Your generation—whatever age you are—did not invent sex. And you probably thought about it whether or not anyone had told you about it. Yet we expect our teenagers, hormones raging and on the threshold of adulthood, to ignore the sexual side of their humanity. Did you, at that age?

Second reality check. When young people are confronted by these powerful feelings and desires but are not given a strong base of knowledge and values that form a context about what saying "yes" means and what saying "no" means, and what constitutes appropriate behavior—well, it stands to reason that some young women will engage in behavior that will not be in their best interest. And even the teenagers who do abstain in their teen years will eventually need these skills—the average person today is sexually active for nine years before marrying in their mid-to-late twenties.

Third reality check. Ignorance is not bliss, but facts alone aren't enough to get teens across the maturation Rubicon. Context is all-important, including practicing decision-making skills, being and feeling valued by parents but also by society, and having solid relationships with responsible adults.

Fourth reality check. Even when we talk to our children about sex, we rarely talk about intimacy, desire, and sexual pleasure. There's a general cultural norm—reinforced by the way we talk to our children when we do talk to them about sex, and by images in the mass media—that males want sex and females want relationships. In reality, both want both and need to learn how to handle both.

But they don't learn what they need to know to handle this need for intimacy or their desires or the experience of sexual pleasure. In a study of students and dropouts in New York City, researchers found that girls' sexuality was generally talked about in terms of victimization, violence, and morality, but rarely in terms of desire. And, the study found, the girls who became pregnant were not necessarily the most overtly sexual, but often those who were most passive and lacking in a sense of personal and sexual self-entitlement. Many are quite conflicted about whether or not to engage in intercourse, and without a strong sense of self-worth, it is very difficult to act from conviction. Combine that with sexual ignorance and you have Caitlyn's story:

 Have you ever been in love? Have you ever thought you were in love? I have and I think I am, I've gone to serious measures to prove my love to a boy. I've been dating this one guy for over a year. We started having sex a few months ago and now all I do is wait and worry that my period will never come. We use condoms and my friend gave me some of her left over packs of birth control pills. Other friends of mine say it is not safe to use another persons pills, but just to feel safe I use them anyway. I'm so confused and I'm so scared. I wish I had never had sex yet. I always thought I would wait until I was married, but I gave it up to a boy who said "I Love You."

The amazing power of choosing

Women of all ages tend to date men who are older. That's not so bad for a thirty-year old, but it creates a dangerous power imbalance for younger women who do not have a strong, positive self-image and the ability to embrace their own sexual power straightforwardly. From her vantage point, now as a nineteen-year-old, Rosario tells her story:

 I was fifteen, unsure of what I wanted but who isn't at fifteen? One night, I decided to go out to a *quincenera*. [She met two brothers, both of whom were attracted to her and took her number.] I ended up talking with the younger of them, and he was nineteen. I fell in love with him. I'd wake him in the morning after being on the phone with him all night. I'd go to school and call him from the pay phone and he'd let me go to class when our two-minute warning bell rang—after school, I had fifteen minutes to go to my locker from one end of campus to the other and walk home and call him. He was always keeping track of me, always jealous, he made me feel desired, needed, wanted, loved . . . he was my first sexual experience/relationship and I was in love and irresponsible. Stupid, huh!!!

Yes, this was yet another fifteen-year-old in love with a nineteen-year-old, and, yes, she became pregnant. She chose not to continue the pregnancy. In my case, abortion was whispered as a possibility (yes, even in those very pre-*Roe* days) but I wanted to have a child. It was my passive, jelly woman way of taking a measure of control over my life, in keeping with my idealized notion of womanhood.

But there is a unifying thread between Rosario's story and mine that happened almost two generations apart. The shame of acknowledging sexual activity outside our parents' and society's expectations of celibacy until marriage was greater than the pain of carrying out a heart-wrenching decision alone and without parental support. I do not know how she felt, but I felt numb, vacant, and it would take many years for me to renew my sense of self as I came first to own, and then to value, the power of choosing.

Breaking the mold by redefining the problem

There are solutions that work to help young people avoid having to make either Rosario's decision or mine, for there are many ways to give children opportunities to grow by making choices. The solutions will require us to change how we talk about sex throughout the diverse cultures represented in our society.

We have only to look at how these issues are handled in Western Europe and Canada to see that something is seriously amiss in the U.S. Here, we tell teens to just say "no." There, they tell them about sex and relationships; they tell them to wait until they are mature enough and ready to accept the consequences. They fortify them with strong decision-making skills based on unvarnished information about what "yes" means, and they tell them how to protect themselves when they become sexually active. All without embarrassment. They assume that young people, girls as well as boys, will eventually have sex, and they treat sexuality as a healthy, normal part of life.

They define the problem as teen pregnancy; we define it as teen sexuality. They see teen pregnancy as a public health problem; we see teen sexuality as a moral problem.

Comprehensive sexuality education in schools is routine in most other industrialized countries, as is affordable and confidential access to family planning services. But there is more to it. A young woman who was an exchange student in the Netherlands told me that parents there seemed to care about the quality of their child's relationships rather than whether or not there was sexual activity. Sex is a good word not a shameful one at home, in school, in the media, and in the culture at large. For both boys and girls.

The results? They have healthy young people and far less unintended pregnancy, abortion, and sexually transmitted infections at all ages. We have a public health crisis of pregnancy and disease. Teen pregnancy is higher in the U.S. than almost any other developed nation—two-to-ten times higher here than in most Western European countries and Canada. We know how to change that and we have made substantial progress—a 20 percent reduction in teen pregnancy during the past decade by employing some of those same techniques in spite of a strident opposition. Ellen's words are testimony to why I have confidence in young people's ability to absorb information and use it intelligently:

 Knowing about pregnancy and sex in general has made me a better teenager. I'm nineteen years old and proud to be a virgin. I planned when I was young to save myself for marriage and I still feel that way.

Shelly, now twenty-seven, looks back on her teen years and offers a prescription for today's teens:

 We need legislators who understand that not every child will be provided with accurate and appropriate sexual health information at home. Although it is ideal for teens to abstain from sex until they are physically and emotionally ready to deal with the consequences, we need legislators who know that many adolescents will not abstain. These teens need to know that their lives are not any less valuable just because they have chosen to have sex. We need schools that provide these teens with the information necessary to keep their bodies safe and healthy.

And Cindy, whose story introduces this "growing up" section said:

 If adults want to lower the rates of problems, they should embrace and praise the teens who actually do have safe sex.

Searching for "h. e. r.": honesty, equality, responsibility

The mind, body, and spirit are enriched by the healthy, responsible enjoyment of sex. We must teach young people exactly what it means to be healthy and responsible about sex. In order to do that, we have to talk to them about it. And we have to show them by our words and our actions that they can come to us for help. We must teach our sons as well as our daughters the importance of honesty, equality, and responsibility in relationships:

 Sometimes the people that feel the loneliest are never actually alone. I spent so much time with my four best friends, it was ridiculous. But I was always so lonely. My parents have always been very involved in their work. And my older brother had moved out. I missed getting attention from them. So, with psychology backing me up, I turned to other males for attention. I started having sex with anyone and everyone. Sex was supposed to connect people. So, whenever I was feeling lonely, I turned to sex in an attempt to connect with someone. It didn't work. I felt horrible about myself, especially because no one had any respect for me anymore. Now I have realized sex won't fill the emptiness in your heart if you do it with people you don't even know well, never mind love. Sex can be a beautiful thing, but if you do it for the wrong reasons, all emotion is lost. It becomes like brushing your teeth. And let's face it; no one would turn to brushing teeth when they are feeling lonely.

—Tamra, age eighteen

 I never let my boyfriend be an influence on me on having sex for the first time. I always felt that being ready was the most important thing. So I waited until I was ready and I discovered that having sex with the right person is the greatest feeling in the world, but only when you are completely ready.

—Kim, age eighteen

Jennifer, whose story appeared earlier in this chapter, now tells the rest of her story.

 I immediately decided that I never wanted to see him again [after the initial bad experience], and that I would not have sex for a very long time.

Now we get to the being ready part. My boyfriend of a year and I began dating last spring, and about six months into the relationship, the topic of sex came up. We sat down together and discussed the pros and cons of it. We also discussed all of the consequences, good or bad, and what we would do about them. Also, he brought up why he wanted to have sex with me. It wasn't because he was a teenage male, or he had a reputation to uphold, he said that it was because he believed that we had something very special together, and he wanted to take the next step with me.

I searched inside myself and tried to find doubts. It was surprising when I found none. I could not think of one reason to not share this experience with him. My gut felt great, and my mind was clear and focused. I was his first, and I wish that he was mine. For anyone that has any doubts about having sex, my advice is wait. I know you've heard it a million times: You'll know when it's the right time, but from experience I can tell you, you'll know when it's the wrong time.

I am convinced that there is one more essential change that must take place if we want strong girls to become strong women, not jelly, when it comes to boys and sex. We must deal with the mold, not just the jelly recipe. We must create a culture in which girls and women are truly valued as much as boys and men. This is the linchpin, when joined with honest information, that can make all the difference in holding together the disparate parts of a girl's developing personality, allowing her to keep her own sense of self:

 I want everyone out there to realize that you don't have to deal with abusive relationships, insensitive partners who make you feel low nor do you have to be the one making all the sacrifices. Breaking off a relationship with someone you love who doesn't treat you right can be very hard, but you'll never regret it. There are thousands of people out there who are looking for someone just like you. And they may be the one that you need to help you appreciate yourself and live out your dreams.

—Jamila, age seventeen

We can walk alongside our daughters as they grow from strong girls to strong women, without that dangerous jelly detour along the way. This young woman tells us how much she appreciates that:

When I was a teen I got involved in a program where we were taught to do a number of things to prepare us for the real world. We were taught to be peer counselors for other teens in the community. We were taught issues concerning AIDS, contraception, sexually transmitted diseases, female and male reproductive system, how to communicate in public effectively. We broadcast a television show concerning issues pertinent to teens and I even got to meet Cecily Tyson. There were so many other helpful topics. That program taught us so many skills that I still use today. The biggest reason to say thank you is because the program taught me not to give in to peer pressure and that it was okay to abstain from sex until we were ready.

—Bree, age twenty

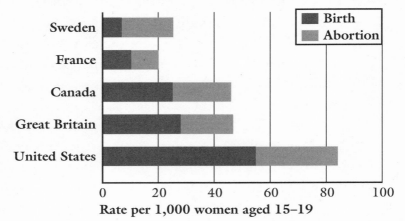

U.S. teenagers have higher pregnancy, birth and abortion rates than adolescents in other developed countries

Legend:
- ■ Birth
- ■ Abortion

Rate per 1,000 women aged 15–19

Note: Data are for mid-1990s.

The Alan Guttmacher Institute, Teenage Sexual and Reproductive Behavior in Developed Countries, *Facts in Brief,* 2001.

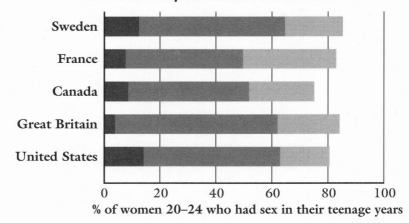

Differences in levels of teenage sexual activity across developed countries are small.

% of women 20–24 who had sex in their teenage years

- ■ By age 15
- ■ By age 18
- ■ By age 20

Note: Data are for mid-1990s.

The Alan Guttmacher Institute, Teenage Sexual and Reproductive Behavior in Developed Countries, *Facts in Brief,* 2001.

What Makes the Difference?

> **Positive attitudes about sexuality and clear expectations for behavior in sexual relationships contribute to responsible teenage behavior.**

- Countries other than the United States have greater openness and more supportive attitudes about sexuality.
- There is a strong consensus in countries other than the United States that childbearing belongs in adulthood.
- Countries other than the United States give clearer and more consistent messages about appropriate sexual behavior.

> **Positive attitudes about sexuality and clear expectations for behavior in sexual relationships contribute to responsible teenage behavior.**

- Comprehensive sexuality education, not abstinence promotion, is emphasized in countries with lower teenage pregnancy levels.
- Media is used less in the United States than elsewhere to promote positive sexual behavior.
  - Government media campaigns in the other countries promote condom use, contraceptive use, and awareness of where to get methods.
  - Media campaigns in other countries offer more positive views of sexually active teenagers as worthwhile, responsible people.

> **Strong and widespread government support for young people's transition to adulthood, and for parents, may contribute to low teenage birthrates.**

- Education and employment assistance help young people become established as parents.
- Support for working parents and families signifies the high value of children and parenting, and gives youth the incentive to delay childbearing.

The Alan Guttmacher Institute. Teenage Sexual and Reproductive Behavior in Developed Countries. *Facts in Brief.* 2001.

Chapter Three

"He told me not to tell."

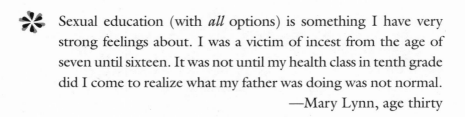 Sexual education (with *all* options) is something I have very strong feelings about. I was a victim of incest from the age of seven until sixteen. It was not until my health class in tenth grade did I come to realize what my father was doing was not normal.

—Mary Lynn, age thirty

Conspiracy of silence and shame

The conspiracy of silence about sex, on both a personal and social level, still leaves girls vulnerable to so many things. Pregnancy and disease, of course. But also exploitation by sexual predators. And they will know, thanks to our silence, that we're not the ones they can come to for help. I find it is extraordinary to read the hundreds of letters from young women and see how many stories contain a thread of sexual abuse. A recent University of Pennsylvania study concludes that sexual abuse of young people is far more common than previously thought— and that we ought to be teaching our children to beware of relatives and friends, who commit nearly all of the abuse, as well as the strangers who are responsible for a small percentage of it.

I knew nothing about sex but I was in trouble because of rape.

—Tameyra, age thirty-eight

 It all started when these two guys from my school found out that I had an eating disorder. I denied it but they knew I was lying and told me that if I didn't let them do what they wanted to do to me then they would tell my parents and I would be put in a hospital. They knew I was *really* scared about that happening . . . I was at a big end-of-the-year party when they pulled me into the garage in the basement and said if I tried to stop them then they would call my mom and tell her about me. I did not know what to do because they had a phone in their hand. They took my shirt and bra off me and then put their hands down my pants. It went on for a while. It was terrible and for a long time after that I wasn't myself. I now know that none of it was my fault and by talking to my friends about it I have gotten over it.

—Joy, age nineteen

Ira Reiss, in *An End to Shame,* estimates that 80 percent of all rapes involve people who know each other—acquaintance and date rape. He attributes this to a traditional view of dating in which the female is expected to be reluctant to have sex and the male is expected to per-suade her otherwise. Because neither party has been taught the com-munications skills that would enable them to talk honestly about their relationship and sexual behavior, they turn to manipulation and clues (did she laugh at a dirty joke?). Because "no" ceases to mean " no" when he believes she will always say "no."

 Raped at age fifteen while still a virgin . . . Got an STD [sexu-ally transmitted disease] check without my mom. I couldn't tell her that her little girl got drunk and date-raped.

—Tisha, age seventeen

I was raped when I was at a party by a guy friend of mine. I was drinking and I passed out and he had sex with me. I woke up crying and sick. My dress was no place to be found and he was still on top of me. Most of the girls took my side but my guy friends took his side. I was called a slut and worse. I didn't tell my parents or the police because I was scared. And now six years later I'm getting past it . . . with the help of my family who now knows.

—Misty, age twenty-three

"It was, after all, my fault."

The sense of responsibility that girls have for the reprehensible behavior of their "partners" in these cases is shocking and sad, as Patty's story illustrates:

 I was fourteen years old and dedicated to the belief that sex should wait for marriage. I had a very close friend who was also my neighbor. All of my friends and I hung out with them and spent lots of time together. One day, my friend who was eighteen, when I was fourteen went *way* too far. I was scared and suddenly I felt a searing pain in my groin. I pushed him off of me but he came back at me. I was crying the whole time. He left me all alone after he was finished raping me. I was so scared and so alone.

Later he called and told me over and over that it was all my fault. He couldn't control himself around me because he "loved" me and I was *so* beautiful. I couldn't bear to tell my mother I was so scared. Soon he made this forceful sex a ritual, all the while I cried and pretended it wasn't happening. After all, he said he loved me and it was "my" fault.

After about a month of this, my mother found him having sex with me. I was relieved but it was so traumatic. She called the police and she beat me and told me I was a whore. To make matters worse, I was pregnant. I told the police that I had consensual sex with my friend just to keep him out of trouble because it was, after all, "my" fault.

As much as we'd like to protect all our children, by the time they are teenagers, they are living in the real world where there are far too many tragic realities, and "yes" and "no" are sometimes truly out of their control. Some lack family support, or even homes to live in.

 I was twelve years old alone on the streets of Washington. I knew the risk of getting raped was there, so I tried to buy condoms . . . they wouldn't let me. I got raped a few days later, I even got pregnant. I went through with it and gave my baby up for adoption when she was two weeks old. That was three years ago and to this day I haven't seen her. It has caused me more grief than anything.

—Renee, age fifteen

 I found out I was pregnant at age sixteen. I was only a kid at the time and I had been raped. I was ashamed because no one I knew would understand.

—Melissa, age thirty-eight

 Thank you teenwire.com for your article on how to help a friend who was raped. My 14-year-old friend was raped by one of her brother's friends. It happened last summer so I didn't really know what to do. I just tried to stay by her side and not talk about it unless she wanted to. Now that I have read this article, I'll know how to handle it when we talk about it next time.

—Angela, age fifteen

 Basically what happened was, I said no and he said yes and that was the end of that. I didn't tell anyone for six months that it had happened, and it really messed my life up. I was ashamed and blaming myself. I thought that I had something to do with it. You don't though. Something such as rape is never anyone's fault but the rapist.

—Lisa, age twenty-two

The conspiracy of ignorance, silence, and shame about sexuality and sexual behavior ratchets up dramatically the difficulty young people have navigating the system to find help when they have been abused or sexually exploited. I found these two stories especially compelling:

 At the age of eleven I was raped by a cruel man and consequently became pregnant. After I had the child I found out that the male doctor who had treated me knew about Emergency Contraception but felt that I was this little girl playing grown-up and when the game became too real for me I cried rape. This man had decided my life when he judged me and took away my right to choose.

 I can relate to the twelve-year-old who was raped by a twenty-year-old. I was raped by someone who forced me to do it twice. I had to deal with the court system and a lot of heartache. The judge only made him serve five years probation and thirty days community service. And the worst part of it all it wasn't his first time preying on young girls my age. It has now been three years since it happened and thank goodness I could get on with my life.

"My alternate plan was suicide."

The greater the difference in age, the greater the power imbalance and the more likely it is that young girls and women will be sexually exploited by older boys and men. It is also more likely that they will not use contraception:

I was fourteen when I found out that I was pregnant. The father was four years my senior and very manipulative. I decided to have an abortion, but the night before my appointment my parents uncovered the truth about my situation. Luckily for me I was still allowed to obtain my abortion. I did, however, lose the respect and admiration of my parents. I can't imagine having a six-year-old right now. I would not be close to my college graduation, have scholarship offers for my master's degree, or probably be alive today (my alternate plan was suicide). Young people need the tools to stop these unwanted pregnancies.

—Elsie, age twenty-one

And puppy love isn't necessarily all it's cracked up to be—teen relationships also hold the possibility of violence and abuse. After all, teens most often model their experience on adult behavior.

 I am a youth advocate and I work in middle schools and high schools in the Midwest. I work in a dating violence prevention program and I primarily work with young women who are already in, or are at high risk for being in a violent relationship. Far too often I encounter adults who simply cannot believe that relationships at this age can ever move past the "puppy love" stage, they simply cannot understand that teen relationships can be as serious as adult relationships with all the same, very real feelings.

—Jason, age nineteen

 Unfortunately my boyfriend was a full-blown alcoholic which I didn't realize until after I'd "fallen in love with him." He would become violent and aggressive on the nights he drank hard. It was easier to just not use a condom than to make him angry. I allowed him to do whatever he wanted to me. I mean, he loved me right? He said he did. But he didn't. He loved having sex with me. He didn't love me. When I found out I was pregnant . . . he asked me if it was his. Of course it was his, but like most other things in his life, he would have rather not had to take responsibility for it. I begged him to come be with me when I got the abortion. He promised, and never came.

—Liz, now twenty-five,
talking about her experience at age eighteen

One-third of women and girls globally will experience some form of abuse in their lives, much of it sexual. In the U.S., one woman in six has experienced some form of sexual abuse. And a history of sexual abuse seems to make it more likely that teens (and adults) will practice risky sexual habits, such as having multiple partners and failing to protect themselves against pregnancy and disease. Jelly women can't confront this, but strong girls will if they have the information, skills, and parental support—and if we can love them enough to allow them access to other institutional help when they can't talk to us. Because sometimes someone in the family is the problem.

"An environment that permits the sexual abuse of a child is not one that fosters open discussion of reproductive health care."

Again, our social schizophrenia toward sexuality is hurting our children. Reiss says that homes where sex is considered dirty, a taboo subject, where the parents have restrictive attitudes toward sex, and fathers feel they have authority over their wives and children, are often backdrops for sexual abuse. I could fill the entire book with stories, but the four letters that follow illustrate the range of experiences suffered by girls who are brought up in these households, whether we want to acknowledge it or not.

 I have had to face a lot in my life and the one bad thing is my uncle molesting my older sister. He meant the world to me and

I never thought that anything like that could ever happen in my family. Now I have no idea what to do about the whole situation, I'm afraid that he will try to come after me. Can someone please help me and tell me what I should do.

—Anonymous question to Web site

 Only a small fraction of rapes are reported to the police. Virtually no incest cases are reported to the police, because the child is threatened with death if they ever tell anyone. I spent a day crying, thinking of all the little girls raped by fathers/stepfathers/uncles/etc. and the hell they must go through if they get pregnant. I was lucky, in a sick sense: my father raped me repeatedly throughout my childhood, but he had a vasectomy before I hit puberty.

—Valerie, age thirty-six

 Sexual health was not openly discussed in my family. As a child, I was sexually abused by my older brother. Despite telling my mother of the abuse after the first incident, it continued for several years. An environment that permits the sexual abuse of a child is not one that fosters the open discussion of reproductive healthcare. I was therefore not taught to respect my body, and for a long time I did not. Had I become pregnant as an adolescent, I don't know that I would have been able to safely seek the support of my parents. I fear for adolescents, living in similar home environments, who may be negatively impacted by parental notification laws.

—Elizabeth, age twenty-seven

We should not be shocked by the revelations that many supposedly celibate priests have a history of sexually abusing minor boys and girls. Nor should we be shocked that it has taken so many years for their stories to come to light. First, these young people are in situations where they are unlikely to have been taught about sex, so how could they possibly know how to protect themselves from inappropriate sexual behavior? Second, they are vulnerable because of the power imbalance between themselves and revered authority figures. A well-informed child is much less likely to be sexually abused. She or he will understand that what is happening is wrong. She or he will have been taught what is appropriate or not and what to do if confronted by inappropriate advances.

Finding the strength to heal

From a child advocate who has seen the devastating results of sexual and other child abuse, and understands the underlying causes:

 When I started practicing law about thirty years ago, I became involved in a *pro bono* project for abused children. Through this work, I became aware that many abused children were children born at the wrong time for their parents, overwhelmingly close in age to their siblings, during periods of financial problems, marital stress, unemployment, or who were unwanted children. It logically followed to me that if women and men could make better choices about their fertility, our children would grow up in safer homes, and in healthier families.

—David, age fifty-five

Sometimes, the young woman does find the strength somewhere, from a supportive adult, an institution that can provide the services she needs to heal and move on, or from the process of her own maturation. When she has been able to avoid unintended pregnancy or childbearing, her chances are much better. The rest of Patty's story (see page 42) is one of those happy endings:

 I am now twenty years old, in school as a premed student and engaged to a wonderful man. I owe my whole future to that abortion. If it wasn't for the choice of abortion, I'd have a five-year-old child and be on welfare with no hope of college. It's not fair to say that abortion should only be legal for rape or incest. Although mine was rape, I didn't put it on record as such. Many young women may be in the same predicament. I'm so glad that I have a promising future. Because of abortion, the world will soon have a new ob/gyn named Dr. Patty Gomez. Abortion should be available for *every* woman to make her own decision, *no matter what!*

During my lifetime, I have seen the very definition of sexual abuse evolve as women have become empowered through reproductive and other civil rights. What I accepted as the norm—the unsolicited pats on the butt, the comments about breast size, the leers and innuendoes about how to get what we want—many women today recognize as harassment or abuse, and I say "go, girls!" But so often, even today, we have to learn the hard way. And far too often, perhaps in direct proportion to the number of jelly woman images and sexual ignorance to which a girl has been acculturated, the crime is neither recognized nor reported until many years later. When the question is sex, our young people need more than silence. They need the information and skills to handle these situations. They need to know that they can come to us for help, and they need to know where they can go for help when one of us is the problem.

Chapter Four
Pierced ears

 When I was seventeen, I went to a local clinic to have an exam, so that I could get a prescription for birth control pills without having to ask my parents. My mom and dad had always stressed to me that I could come to them about sexual matters and were open with me about sex; they even contributed both their time and money to Planned Parenthood! But still, for whatever reason, I felt like this was something I wanted to do on my own.

—Andrea, age twenty-two

Minors do consent

I don't have pierced ears. I figure that if God had wanted us to have holes in our ears, she would have put them there. So when my daughters, aged eleven and thirteen and generally well behaved, wanted to get their ears pierced, I said no. Soon after, my daughter Linda and a friend went into the bathroom and with a sterilized needle and ice as anesthetic, pierced each other's ears. They did a pretty good job of it, too. They unwittingly, or maybe wittingly, taught me that there is a big difference between parental authority in theory—where the rules are made—and in the real world. Yes, they needed my consent to have their ears professionally pierced. But just as my daughter and her friend went on to do it themselves, today, without our permission, our adults-in-training are making adult-type decisions about sex.

Because they can, and do, have sex without our consent or knowledge, the issue of their access to the related health care is an important one. This issue was on the agenda at the very first board meeting I attended at Permian Basin Planned Parenthood in 1971 in Odessa, Texas. The board members argued long and loudly about whether to require parental consent for a minor to get birth control. They reached a very foolish compromise to dispense birth control to teenagers who already had what they called an "illegitimate" child. Whereupon the wise county judge, a board member on the losing side of the vote, exclaimed, "Now if that ain't shuttin' the barn door after the cow's got out!"

The debate continues to rage in Congress and state legislatures. The resulting social policy often deals with parent-child relationships concerning sexual matters, not with supportive services and compassion, but with punitive legislation that fruitlessly attempts to force communication in the least appropriate situations.

When we mandate parental consent by law for birth control or abortion, we do not achieve the laudable goal of improving family communication. Instead, we rob our teenagers of the opportunity to take responsibility for their sexual health: something they genuinely want to do, and we put them at great risk of harm. Let's pay attention to these teenagers who could, and did, make their own decisions about birth control. Some of them speak from their now-adult vantage point. Eleven stories follow, but I could have included eleven hundred, all echoing the same theme:

 My parents would kill me if they knew I was having sex. At least this way I'm protected and I feel like I'm being responsible. When the time comes to tell them I can at least say I was protected the whole time and I can choose to tell them myself instead of them finding out cause I'm pregnant.

—Megan, age fifteen

My first visit to a clinic was when I was fifteen. I was thinking about becoming sexually active with my boyfriend. I wanted to be smart about it but I also know there was no way I could tell my folks. Therefore I probably wouldn't be able to afford services. They've always worked around my financial situations and I don't know what I'd do without them.

—Beth, age eighteen

I have been living on my own since I was seventeen. Without birth control I don't know what I would have done. I am one of the few girls I know who hasn't had an abortion.

—Sara, age nineteen

I first came to the clinic at age sixteen when I didn't feel comfortable talking to my mother about birth control. Because they helped me afford the pill, I have not gotten pregnant, and I am able to keep from getting pregnant until marriage. If I had not been given low-cost pills at such a young age I may have gotten pregnant and had to drop out of school rather than becoming a responsible adult who made it through high school and college.

—Katie, age twenty-five

A young girl raised a strict Catholic well, my parents would have never consented to birth control. The clinic not only helped me without my parents consent but counseled me on all facets of sexuality.

—Rita, age twenty-seven

✻ I was sixteen, it was impossible to ask my mom to take me to my gynecologist for birth control. So I dredged up the courage to go to an unfamiliar part of town, wondering whether or not I should give my real name, and walking out happy to have my very own diaphragm. A few years later, I drove my younger sister to the same place for her first birth control.

—Cherie, mid-thirties

✻ The clinic is a way for me to get the health care I need. I like the fact that it is confidential because it made me feel that I had somewhere I could go when I did not feel comfortable talking to my parents about it.

—Cynthia, age twenty

✻ I recently became a "sexually active teen." Of course, my parents are not aware of this. I am aware of the responsibilities that come with sexual intercourse, and the clinic helped me to tend to these responsibilities without being ostracized from my parents. I am glad for this service. If it did not exist, I would not be able to learn how to take care of myself now that I am sexually active (since talking about these things is considered taboo in my culture.)

—Anh, age eighteen

✻ My parents are not supportive or even very willing to discuss sex or reproductive health with me. This is founded in their religious background; a demand for me to remain a virgin until I am married. The clinic has helped me with many things: birth control (affordable), cryotherapy, and many kind and informative words. Without them, I don't know what my life would be like now.

—Rachel, age eighteen

People, as young as I was when I first came here, can know that there is somewhere they can go if they need the services a clinic provides. I started coming when I was 16 and they provided birth control and services that helped me at the time. Teenagers are scared to tell their parents about their sex lives and being able to take care of themselves keeps them from getting pregnant.

—Heidi, age nineteen

 I've been coming to a clinic since I was seventeen. I couldn't talk to my parents about wanting to go on birth control, but I knew the clinic could provide all the important services I needed without parental consent. This helps kids like me make decisions that are positive and affect our entire lives. Nobody wants an unwanted baby in the world.

—Kristen, age twenty-two

Each of these young women, and thousands and thousands of others who use family planning services on their own consent, has achieved what her parents most likely would agree is an admirable goal: she's not pregnant. And she doesn't have to face the difficult decision that comes with an unintended pregnancy.

Not one state requires parental consent for a teenager to receive prenatal care and give birth, or requires parental notification of a teen's positive pregnancy test. All but five allow her to surrender a child for adoption without parental involvement. No state requires parental consent for a minor to get testing and treatment for sexually transmitted infections. The U.S. Supreme Court has extended the right of privacy to use birth control to teenagers, saying the state cannot restrict their access to contraception in order to try to limit their sexual activity. Justice John Paul Stevens said it was like "dramatiz[ing] its disapproval of motorcycles by forbidding the use of safety helmets." Many states have supported that view with their own legislation.

What restricting minors' access is really about

Yet at this writing, forty-two states have passed laws requiring parental notification or consent for abortion, although some of these laws are under court challenge and are not yet enforced. How do they deal with the unfortunate reality that not every teen can talk to her parents? Usually by forcing her to go through a complicated, intimidating judicial process where a judge, not someone who knows her and loves her like an aunt or grandparent, determines whether she is competent to make her own decision. Why are these laws so easy to pass? Because they give otherwise moderate legislators a way to temporarily silence the vocal anti-choice minority while telling the rest of us that the issue isn't abortion, it's the rights of parents to supervise the actions of their children.

Make no mistake—*it is about abortion*. It's just a lot easier for those who oppose abortion to restrict access for the less powerful among us than to outlaw all abortion. It certainly isn't about what's best for minors. Everyone agrees that it's best when teens involve their parents in such decisions, and carry them out with their love and support. Most teens do, especially young teens, and minor teens in families where they can safely communicate with their parents. It isn't about parental rights either. Law and reason have long acknowledged that when teens are sexually active, something they are without parental consent, they need confidential access to related health services. So it doesn't make sense that there is such a ruckus about minors' access to abortion when they have full access to other options with equally profound influence and risks to their lives. Imagine, if you will, that laws required parental consent for a teen to exercise her other option and she had to go to court if she wanted to continue the pregnancy because her parent refused to agree to her prenatal care.

Richard North Patterson, whose bestseller *Protect and Defend* focuses in part on this issue, summed it up nicely in a speech to the National Abortion Rights Action League: "Never addressed is the question of why a minor too immature to decide for herself is nonetheless suited to motherhood."

Nor is the trend to limit minors' access to abortion about supporting families in crisis. Consent laws intrude upon families at the worst possible time and provide no support system to help them cope.

Laws that deny minors' access to abortion are predicated on the misguided notion that if parents knew, they wouldn't let their daughters have abortions. In fact, the contrary just may be true. Ask the people who counsel young women with unintended pregnancies about their options of abortion, adoption, or parenting, they see many more parents who are trying to force their daughters to have abortions than they do ones who are trying to talk them out of it. When I finally told my parents about my situation, it wasn't because a law required me to. And ironically in my state, as in many states, becoming married automatically "emancipates" a minor and empowers her to give legal consent. How did being married suddenly make her into an adult?

 Considering my age, I was a baby, a child. How could I have dealt with my pregnancy then? With what little knowledge I had about teenage pregnancy I knew that I wanted the right to turn my life around in another direction. I was afraid of telling my mother. My mother is a strong advocate for pro-life and adoption. I know had there been a parental consent law in effect I would have given birth at the age of fourteen. I am a struggling college student now and I value all of life's choices and now I have the power to do anything.

—Dawn, age twenty-four

Why some teens don't tell their parents

Why don't some teens involve their parents? Well, if they remain pregnant, eventually they will be helped by nature to deliver the message. Recently, my daughter returned from her high school reunion where she learned that a classmate has a daughter who is a junior in high school and just gave birth. The family had not known she was pregnant until a week before she delivered, thus illustrating that both parents and young people can live in a world of denial and fantasy. Yes, even in the twenty-first century. That denial and terror about owning up to parents about sex and pregnancy, so prevalent in my youth, hasn't fully abated. If minors don't want to remain pregnant, parental involvement laws force them to own up, and owning up means admitting sexual activity.

But there are other legitimate and heart-wrenching reasons that teens do not reveal their pregnancies to their parents. One-third of teens who don't tell have suffered physical or sexual abuse at the hands of their parents and have well-founded fears that the abuse will escalate if the pregnancy is discovered. Some teens fear they'll be kicked out of the house; some have been warned they definitely will be kicked out of the house. Others live with unsupportive relatives or with parents who abuse drugs or alcohol.

The young women who do not tell their parents have such strong reasons for not doing so that these laws are meaningless. The same percentage of teens in states with such laws involve at least one parent in their decision making as do those who live in states *without* consent laws. And in countries where minors can get confidential treatment paid for by government health insurance, the abortion rates are the among lowest in the world.

The counselors who help these young women and the attorneys who see them through daunting judicial bypass proceedings will tell you that the women emerge from these problematic families with the maturity to consider their situations and make the right choice for themselves about an unintended pregnancy.

Joseph Feldman, who has counseled Arizona teens seeking judicial waivers, says that the ability to think realistically about the future, hold a job, and be active in school and at church, accept responsibility at home, volunteer, and have plans for after high school all show the maturity to make an informed decision about an unwanted pregnancy.

"A junior in high school who already wants to go to college and major in biology shows a higher level of maturity than a kid who says 'I don't know, I'll figure it out later.'" In Feldman's experience, the more mature a younger teen is, the more likely it is she will choose abortion when she is fourteen or fifteen years old, while "the teen who can't see the future just thinks she's going to have a baby and everything's going to be cool."

And as we know from the days when abortion was illegal, a woman who has decided that abortion is the best answer for her will go to astonishing lengths to obtain one, risking her health and even her life in the process. Feldman said that not one of the teens who came to him in preparation for going to court for the judicial bypass necessary if a teen needs to circumvent parental consent laws ever backed out. "My perception is that they are generally up to the challenge of going to court" once they have decided that they want to have an abortion and, for whatever reason, can't tell a parent.

Becky Bell, Spring Adams, and other victims of the law

When young women can't legally act without parental consent, tragedy can result. Becky Bell was a seventeen-year-old Indiana girl, a good student who had a warm, open relationship with her parents. But when she became pregnant, she desperately wanted to avoid disappointing them—so desperately that she found a way to get an illegal abortion when a legal one wasn't available to her without her parents' involvement. Like so many women who have turned to the back alley, she faced serious complications after the abortion. Her last words were, "Mom. Dad, I love you. Forgive me." Moments later she died in her parents' arms. Her parents, former supporters of parental consent laws, now speak passionately and publicly against them. And these laws continue to do harm while helping no one.

Thanks to Idaho law, thirteen-year-old Spring Adams had to tell her mother she was pregnant and wanted an abortion. The night before her appointment, her father, who was responsible for her pregnancy, found out. He shot her to death and killed her mother and himself.

A Massachusetts teen going through the court process to get an abortion without consent lost her confidentiality when her sister's civics class paraded through the courthouse.

One of the first teens required to notify her parents under Colorado's law was kicked out of the house and her mother took the money she had saved for the abortion. When the teen was finally able to schedule her appointment, she was living in a friend's car.

Society's skewed view of a thirteen-year-old boy versus a seventeen-year-old girl

In a society where a thirteen-year-old boy can be tried for a crime as an adult because it is believed he can understand the consequences of his actions, a seventeen-year-old girl has to get her parent's permission for abortion because it is believed she can't understand her options. And one of those options is to become a mother at seventeen, incurring tremendous physical, emotional, educational, economic, and social costs.

The teen years are fraught with uncertainties as teens struggle to develop an identity apart from their parents. The importance of parental values can't be overestimated—nor can the importance of providing young people safe harbors in which to practice their decision skills. The reality is that nearly two-thirds of young women seeking an abortion involve at least one parent, and more than half of teens on birth control will eventually confide in a parent. But they don't do it because of some law. The problem is—where does that leave the ones who don't feel they can consult their parents?

Things could get worse. Congress is considering a law that would make it a crime for an adult who is not the parent to take a minor across state lines for the purpose of having an abortion—again, an easy out for legislators who can wave the flag of parental rights. But the Rev. Katherine Hancock Ragsdale, an Episcopal priest from Massachusetts, tried to set them straight. Here are some excerpts from her testimony before the House Judiciary Committee in September 2001:

 I recall vividly a day when I left my home near Cambridge, Massachusetts, and drove to one of the economically challenged cities to the north of me to pick up a fifteen-year-old girl and drive her to Boston for an eight A.M. appointment for an abortion. I didn't know the girl—I knew her school nurse. The nurse had called me a few days earlier to see if I knew where she might find money to give the girl for bus fare to and cab fare home from the hospital. I was stunned—a fifteen-year-old girl was going to have to get up at the crack of dawn and take multiple buses to the hospital alone? The nurse shared my concern but explained that the girl had no one to turn to. She feared for her safety if her father found out and there was no other relative close enough to help. So I went. And during our hour-long drive to Boston we talked.

She told me about her dreams for the future—all the things she thought she might like to do and be. I talked to her about the kind of hard work and personal responsibility it would take to get there. She told me about the guilt she felt for being pregnant—even though the pregnancy was the result of a date rape. She didn't call it that. She just told me about the really cute guy from school who seemed so nice and about how pleased she was when he asked her out. She figured the fault was hers for not somehow having known that he wasn't really the "nice boy" he had seemed.

Although New Hampshire was closer to that girl's home than Boston, as it happened, I did not take her across state lines. Nor did I, to my knowledge, break any laws. But if either of those things had been necessary in order to help her, I would have done them. I have no choice because some years ago I stood before an altar and a Bishop and the people of God and vowed . . . to love and serve the people among whom I work. We are appalled at the thought of any girl having to face and make such a decision without the help of her parents, as well we should be. That is, I have to assume, the noble motive behind this bill. But this is not a bill about solutions; it's a bill about punishments.

Several years ago the Episcopal Church passed a resolution opposing any parental consent or notification requirements that did not include provision for nonjudicial bypass. In our view, any morally responsible notification or consent requirement had to allow young women to turn for help to a responsible adult other than a parent or a judge—to go instead to a grandparent or an aunt, a teacher or neighbor, a counselor, minister, or rabbi. Our resolution encourages the very things this bill would outlaw. We know that no one can simply legislate healthy communication within families. And we know that, of those girls who do not involve their parents, many feared violence or being thrown out of their home. Statistical and anecdotal evidence demonstrates that, in far too many American homes, such fears are not unfounded. There is no excuse good enough to justify legislation or regulation that further imperils young people who are already living in danger in their own homes.

Even if we were to find ourselves drained of the last vestiges of our compassion there would still be a self-interested reason to fear and oppose this legislation. It imperils all young women, even those in our own families. Should Becky Bell have talked to her parents? I think so. Did she exercise poor judgment? Absolutely. But, sisters and brothers, I'm here to tell you, teenagers will, from time to time, exercise poor judgment. It's a fact of nature and there is no law you can pass that will change that. The penalty should not be death. Oppose this bill. Oppose it because no matter how good the intentions of its authors and supporters, it is, in essence, punitive and mean-spirited. Oppose it out of compassion for those young people who cannot, for reasons of their safety, comply with its provisions. If all else fails, oppose it for purely selfish reasons. Oppose it because you don't want your daughter or granddaughter or niece to die just because she couldn't face her parents, and you had outlawed all her other options.

Tragic realities

Becky Bell's tragedy occurred in a functional family. In a family with a history of violence, or where the young woman lives in fear, as did the girl Rev. Ragsdale assisted, or where a family member is a sexual predator, as in Spring Adams' case, or where the parents aren't capable of parenting, consent requirements present almost insurmountable barriers—to the detriment of the physical and mental health of the young woman. Here are some typical cases:

 At the age of seventeen I became pregnant and I have a very strict family who I couldn't dare tell. My best friend brought me to a clinic and I was counseled and I had a termination. It's not something I am proud of but I just wasn't ready for a baby. I now come here every year for oral contraceptives to prevent that from happening again.

—Jerry Lynn, age twenty-five

 I started coming to a clinic when I was seventeen years old. I had family problems. There was no communication between my parents and I. Due to this many of my questions were left unanswered. Being a teenager these days is stressful enough, and being alone with the stresses of sex and pregnancy can be hell. The clinic is a place where women can get questions answered, medical treatment that is vital, and the support that is needed when facing difficult issues such as sex, STDs, pregnancy, and even counseling on family problems . . . much needed assistance to women of all ages, especially teenage girls.

—Ady, age unknown

 Well my story begins in a small trailer park where I lived with my grandma because my parents were to strung out on drugs to care for me. I was fifteen years old. I met a guy that was so nice to me, treated me like a queen or that is what I thought, but he sold and took a lot of drugs and he got me into that stuff pretty deep. We spent all of our time together and I soon dropped out of school. Then I find out I am pregnant! I knew that I couldn't keep a baby in the situation I was in, and adoption was out of the question just because I wasn't willing to quit the drugs and there was no way I would bring a baby into the world like that. So I decided on abortion. It wasn't the greatest experience in the world but my life would have been so hard if I would've kept the baby. I now have a two-year-old daughter and am happily married. This is the way it should have happened the first time but it didn't and I am thankful for my freedom to choose. A woman knows when she is ready, and accidents happen, and that is why we need the right to make decisions about our bodies.

—Hillary, age twenty-eight

Support, not punishment, needed

The sexual abuse she endured as a child—in her own home—shaped Amy's strong feelings about sex education and parental consent laws:

 We need schools that provide accurate sexual health education. Beginning in kindergarten, we need to be taught that we have the right and responsibility to protect our own well being. We need to know that we can assert who can and cannot touch our bodies. Perhaps an environment that promotes an open discussion of sexual health will enable abused children to seek the help of trusted adults. The secrecy surrounding the discussion of sexuality adds to the conspiracy of silence connected to sexual abuse.

We need legislators that realize that communication cannot be mandated. Most children who grow up in healthy home environments will seek the support of their families when making a decision regarding their sexual health. However, children who grow up in unsafe homes should not be punished as a result. We need legislators that realize the potential dangers of parental notification laws. We need to be taught that we have the right, the ability, and the authority to make appropriate decisions concerning our bodies . . . and we need legislative measures that support these rights.

Instead of rigid laws, we need to ensure that supportive counseling is available to teens and their families, together and separately; that medically accurate, comprehensive sexuality education in the schools and in the home teaches young people about their sexual health; that they are taught with a positive, not punitive approach that gives teenagers and their families a safety hatch when they can't cope.

As the bumper sticker says, "If you can't trust me with a choice, how can you trust me with a child?" It is worth restating that no state requires parental consent for a teenager to give birth.

Part II
Choosing a life

I was sixteen then and irresponsible, so much the child I believed I wasn't. I was young, alone, without financial or moral support, and yes I had an abortion. I paid dearly for my ignorance. In those weeks prior to my decision I was presented with a crossroad. On one hand I could carry the pregnancy to term, feel what it truly means to have created a life so sweet and innocent. On the other, to take responsibility for that life. To comprehend that being a creator means being accountable for commitment and should be assumed with sober honesty regarding another's entire existence and welfare.

I made my choice, and I would change nothing. Indeed, I will one day leave this world for the next and I will ask my maker's forgiveness regarding many things, but preventing the birth of a child I had no way of providing for, will not be one of them. Those who have not been in my shoes cannot begin to comprehend the battle that was warring within me. I didn't know what it was to truly be a woman until I was asked to give up the one thing that defines and unites us as a sex. That was the hardest thing I ever had to do. Who am I? I am your daughter. I am your best friend. I am your neighbor, your sister, your wife, your future mother. And I have a story.

—Mandy, age thirty-four

Chapter Five

Jelly woman to handsome princess

 Twenty-two. College graduation right around the corner. Having trouble with the pill, no steady boyfriend, decided to discontinue the pill. Old boyfriend renewed his interest and didn't listen to "be careful, use a condom . . . " I should have been more adamant. He didn't stick around much longer after that anyhow. Never have I hesitated since to stand up for my own well being.

I strongly believe I made the right decision to discontinue the pregnancy. There was no way I could have appropriately provided for a child had the pregnancy continued. I must confess, however, that there are times I ponder just what that 15-year-old would be like today . . . but only for a moment. Just long enough to know that I was lucky to have a choice in the first place and that making a mistake shouldn't mean having a child out of guilt. It shouldn't mean creating a situation where a child feels this guilt and possible resentment; or where a child does not receive all the care it deserves. Healthy adults are the by-products of healthy children. There is already enough unhealthiness in our world. I made the right choice not to contribute to it!

I now have two wonderful stepchildren and a beautiful daughter of my own. I am doing my best to provide them with better tools than I had when it comes to their sexuality, being safe and careful. An essential part of my message to them about such issues is helping them to understand what "having a choice" means. I am confident they are listening . . .

—Leah, late thirties

Standing up for our own well-being

When I look back at my own life, I have to ask myself who was that fifteen-year-old who thought she was all grown up and ready to become a wife and mother? At what point did the child, who placed her chair in the doorway after family dinners so she could hear both the men's political and business conversations in the living room and the women's more personal conversations in the dining room, melt into a teenager who aspired only to be popular and fit in? What was the nexus that made my strength of spirit leave just as the hormones started raging? Where did "I" go? How could I have been so strong and willful with my family, announcing my pregnancy and life's course in no uncertain terms, and so weak and ready to forgo my own intelligence and identity with my peers? Did I really think that my nineteen-year-old boyfriend of three months was my handsome prince? Did I really believe in handsome princes?

Or was I like the thousands of women whose letters fill my files, women of all ages who use the phrase, "I found myself pregnant." We don't say, "I wanted to have sex because it felt good, so I did and then I got pregnant." We say, "I found myself pregnant." As if to say, I was swept away. I had nothing to do with it. I was disembodied from my own sexuality. I was disembodied from my own self. We are disembodied from ourselves.

In *Reviving Ophelia,* psychologist Mary Pipher describes the jelly woman phenomenon when she observes that girls are rewarded for being what the culture wants them to be, not what they may want to be themselves. "Girls are trained to be less than who they really are . . . to sacrifice their true selves." This is particularly true in the experience of sexual desire.

Why sexual and reproductive rights are fundamental

The move from fairy-tale romances to mature relationships can be a difficult one for many women. To make the journey, girls and young women need good role models of adult relationships; the self-esteem and skills to say "no" to sex—and to say "yes," for the right reasons at the right time; the emotional maturity to resist relationships of unequal power or that show signs of becoming abusive. We need to be taught to appreciate sexuality as a positive good for ourselves, not just a way of giving pleasure to someone else. We need positive images of our bodies, and we need to develop and value our own physical as well as emotional strength. I was stunned, for example, when I started lifting weights, to realize how little upper body strength I had and what a difference it made in my self-image to have a little bit of muscle.

Girls and women of all ages need hope for the future, goals for the kind of life they want to lead, and a vision of their own potential. More than anything, they need laws and a culture that elevate women's concerns, including sexual and reproductive rights, to the same level as other fundamental human and civil rights. We fall short on many counts. Gail, now thirty, recounts her story:

 Boys, Dating, Romance, "Love." . . . I was a happy, fun-loving, eighteen-year-old who thought I was immortal. My boyfriend was the "love" of my life. I believed everything that he told me. No matter how outrageous. I had dreams of marrying him. My life, I thought, was perfect. After awhile my relationship became abusive. However, like so many of the abused I believed it was my fault. When I found out I was pregnant, I was unbelievably frightened. My boyfriend disappeared.

Her family was supportive as long as she continued the pregnancy:

 I knew deep in my heart that I could not do this. I left home and stayed with my grandmother who is the first person who spoke with me about abortion. I decided that was the responsible choice. My family did not speak to me for over a year. They told everyone they knew that I was a murderer. That's when I decided women should not be ridiculed and judged because of their choice of what to do with their body. I am married now, with a beautiful daughter.

Marcie's story shows that as she puts it, "Real life isn't much like a fairy tale," and that women of all ages need a supportive culture that respects their choices:

 At thirty-four, supporting my two boys and an alcoholic husband, I recently became pregnant. . . . I had the financial means and the experience to care for another baby. But I could not bring another child into an already unstable home and further cement myself and my kids into a bad relationship. This decision has allowed me the opportunity to get my life back on track again, and more, has positively impacted the lives of my sons.

We use the power we have to find purpose and meaning

Pregnancy can be a show of sexual power, of adult power, especially for adolescents. Indeed, it can be the only female power that is rewarded. More often than we ever admit, a pregnancy crisis at any age can return jelly women to the strength of their preadolescent, independent spirits and propel them onward to become strong, mature women. Choosing in and of itself is empowering, whatever the choice. When we as women can be honest about our sexual behavior, reproductive choices, and their consequences, we have a better chance at defining our own futures. Dr. Alfredo Vigil, a New Mexico physician, shared with me elements of this phenomenon within his Hispano culture:

 For a young woman, say in her late teens, with mediocre or poor grades, there is not much of a future to look forward to. But by becoming a mother she is suddenly the center of attention—a wonderful baby shower will likely be thrown by her friends and relatives. She will probably be eligible for Medicaid and other benefits that might actually be better than the benefits available through employer-provided health insurance. There will be much planning for the birth. After the birth the extended family and friends will all visit and congratulate mom with offers of love and support. Grandma and *tias* will be available to baby-sit and help with raising the baby in many ways. In short, life will now have purpose and meaning.

Purpose and meaning. Here are the first-person stories of a variety of young women who faced unintended pregnancies and related how this crisis influenced their lives as they sought their own purpose and meaning through the process of choosing a path.

 We were stupid, we stopped using birth control, and I got pregnant. I cannot afford having a baby, I don't want kids right now, I'm not sure if I could handle a pregnancy emotionally, and I couldn't face having a child only to give it up. A few of my friends have had babies and kept them. They love their kids like nothing else, but the situations they are in are unstable. I really like my situation in life right now. I'm not ready to take the next step, the family step. And, seeing my friends' lives, it seems like having kids at nineteen, twenty, or even earlier leaves you with a lack of self-empowerment.

—Emily, age twenty-one

 I am an eighteen-year-old mother, I have a two-year-old son named Malcolm. For the past three years, I have dropped out of school, started working full time at a retail store, worked until my ninth month of pregnancy, and then gave birth to my beautiful little boy. From that point on, I have realized the things that I then needed to do, not only for my son, but for myself. I went back to school, worked a part-time job, and did the best I could raising my son. I became the student body president, my senior year, and took accelerated classes. I went on to graduate at the top of my class, with honors. Though I didn't get to go to a junior or senior prom, I have enjoyed raising my son. I just want kids to know that if you have the choice to have safe and protected sex, then why don't you take that choice? I made the choice not to, and am now living the life of an adult.

—Leah, age eighteen

 I was in my freshman year of college at the time, in the midst of youthful experimentation. My suite mate's boyfriend was visiting with his friend, and we did what most college kids do— went drinking. Well, after three frat parties, we all stumbled back to the suite. I was half conscious, but vaguely remember my friend's boyfriend's friend coming in my room with me. Through periodic blackouts, I realized what was going on, but was too drunk to stop it. The next morning, they left. I felt so dirty, and vowed never to have sex again. A month later, I was late and I knew exactly why. The test confirmed my worst fear. I immediately made an appointment, and that was the turning point in my life. I never heard from or saw that guy again.

Imagine if I'd had his baby? What would I tell the child about its father? Thank god I was able to make that choice. What life would that baby have had? An alcoholic eighteen-year-old mother who wouldn't even take care of her self, and no father to speak of. I know one day I will have kids, and I will be educated, responsible and have a wonderful father figure for them. This is why we need to make sure every woman has that choice of "someday", but that day will be up to them.

—Kiersten, age twenty-three

 I never had an abortion but I am pro-choice for those out there who became pregnant because their self-esteem was so low they were afraid to say "no," didn't have facts, couldn't speak to their parents, afraid of conditional love from their parents, or were forced to have sex.

—Alice, age thirty

The real sexual revolution and its biological antecedents

Let's face it—we're not all going to be celibate during the years between puberty and marriage. In fact, few of us will be.

Throughout most of human history, puberty and marriage happened about the same time, in the mid-to-late teens. Thanks to improved nutrition and health care, puberty now usually occurs in the preteen years. And due to the need for more and more education in order to make it in our complex society, marriage is delayed until the mid-twenties. That gives the average young woman and man thirteen years of physical maturity between puberty and marriage.

The advent of the birth control pill in 1960 profoundly changed the gender power-balance by allowing women to control their own fertility effectively, pick and choose their partners, and choose to marry or not. The freedom of separating sex from procreation—traditionally granted only to men—marked the true sexual revolution. But this revolution is about much more than sex. It places women on an equal footing with men for education, employment, and other life aspirations. That's why it is possibly the most significant advance in social justice and women's health in human history.

The timing of puberty, marriage, and childbearing has changed, but that doesn't mean that attitudes have kept pace. All too often, rational discussions of sex and sexuality are drowned out by the strident voices of those who fear anything that allows women to act with moral autonomy—and those voices are not just male voices. This culturally ingrained hostility to women won't go away by itself. Some women even want the benefit of gender equality without the burden of the battles that brought us this far. That's why we still hear jelly woman statements like, "I'm not a feminist, but . . ."

Putting jelly woman aside: "a new look in my eye"

Somewhere through the early adult years, I hope, most of us do put aside jelly woman, who knows only how to be "swept away," and gain the inner strength that allows us to make our own decisions about having sex, or not, with whom and for what reasons.

 The first thing to sex is having that talk with your partner. If that doesn't work out, it probably won't work out in bed either.

—Laurie, age twenty-four

 I became an advocate for reproductive choice because growing up, I saw that being able to control my fertility was the first step in having control over my life. By controlling if and when to have children, I could determine whether I lived a life that would be better than my parents or whether it would be marred by poverty, unfulfilled ambitions and a limited education. I grew up in the neighborhood of Washington Heights in New York City which was, and still is predominantly Dominican and poor. Growing up as a Dominican-American woman, it was drilled into me that being a wife and mother was the sole purpose of my existence, but I knew that if I were to thrive instead of merely survive, I needed to focus on getting an education.

All of my life I grew up watching girls as young as twelve and thirteen having babies, dropping out of school, barely surviving on welfare only to watch their own children repeat the same history. It disturbed me to see so many bright and funny girls [become] young women struggling to raise their children and taking their frustration out on them, not for lack of love, but because they are so utterly ill-equipped to handle the stress of raising their children with such limited resources. My own aunt was fourteen when she had her first child. By the time she was twenty-five, she had had four children, one of which was born prematurely because she had developed an addiction to heroin while he was in utero. Out of these four children, one has served time in prison, one became a teen parent herself, one has significant developmental problems and one is successful. My aunt died of AIDS at the age of forty-three. I miss her. And I often wonder how her life might have turned out (and the life of her children) if she had been informed of the reproductive options in her life and encouraged to use them.

I believe that it has been the constant reminder of watching these young women struggle and the memory of my aunt's life that has motivated me to be so vocal about reproductive choice and motivated me to finish my degree at Columbia University. I want Latina girls to know that they have reproductive choices and that they have every right to exercise them and to thrive.

—Estelle, age thirty-five

 I came home from college for break and my mother saw a strange, new "look" in my eyes, on my face, my aura gave me away— *something*. She asked *no* questions, but packed me up and took me to a clinic for an examination and pills. . . . By the way, she was absolutely *correct* about what she saw on my face (smile)!!!

—Brenda, fifties

Choosing wisely

And here's what the world looks like when the principles of honesty, equality and responsibility inform our relationships. I was privileged to know the late Pat Geiser, described by her son Jim in the letter below. She devoted her life to bettering the lives of women everywhere.

 Many years ago, our parents did something only a few married couples did then and almost no one does now. They *planned* their marriage, not just their wedding! Father would finish college while Mother worked. They would delay starting their family for a while. When they did have children, they would have only as many as they believed they could properly raise, based on their realistic projections of their intellectual, emotional, spiritual, social, physical and financial resources.

Linda, who tells how she is raising her child, could also be a role model for women with sons:

 I am thirty-seven years old, married, and a mother of one. I would like my son to know that he was wanted. I want my son to know that my husband and I waited years to have him because we were not ready. I want my son to know that his father and I shared in birth control responsibilities. I want my son to know that his father cared that birth control pills could be bad for me. I want my son to know that his father says that wearing a condom doesn't really change how sex feels for a man. I want my son to know that men want women to have the right to choose what happens with their bodies. I want my son to choose wisely.

Our modern contraceptive methods have given us freedom of choice. But technology doesn't necessarily change values and the larger culture in which our relationships are formed. That's a far more complicated process, fraught with pain as well as gain for all concerned.

There are advantages to being jelly woman, after all. You don't have to take responsibility for your actions, since they were merely reactions. Life can be much less complicated when someone else is making choices for you. And maybe you think you've found a handsome prince who's more than a fairy tale, and you want to believe he'll take care of you for the rest of your life. Or maybe your handsome prince has convinced you to work outside the home, when you want to be home with the kids—or vice versa. Does today's jelly woman want a man to take care of her material needs, maybe in backlash against feminism or out of fear of the responsibilities that freedom brings?

My personal journey from jelly woman to handsome princess and butterfly days

I remember well the moment I decided that I am the handsome princess and I can and should take care of myself. My then-husband earned a stable salary, often working two jobs to support the family's basic needs. (After all, men who become fathers while in their teens don't have it so easy, either.) After our third child was born, a few days after my twentieth birthday, a light bulb went off in my head. I realized that if I had to support those three children, I would be up a creek because I had no employable skills. I headed to the local community college.

I called my father and asked for the one hundred dollars I needed for my first classes, and he happily obliged. After that, I was able to get small scholarships to pay for my tuition. It took me twelve years to finish my bachelor's degree, partly for lack of funds, partly because I made sure to minimize the time I spent away from the children, and partly because I worked part of the time to supplement the family income. As the children grew, their needs grew with them. I wanted them to have music lessons and such, and the simple demands of things like Pop Warner football and band camp were multiplied by three.

Surprise—I liked having money that I had earned, and I liked adding to the family income. I liked the sense of accomplishment for work well done. I aspired to get my teaching credentials so I could earn more than I was making at Head Start where I had begun to work part-time. That alone was a huge step. I was still a traditional wife and "supermom" in addition to holding a job and going to school.

After eleven years of plugging away, I found that a group of beige trailer houses set on a dusty field of newly seeded Bermuda grass east of town were my salvation. The new University of Texas Permian Basin (UTPB) opened in the fall of 1973 as an upper division undergraduate and graduate school. Hot dog. I could finish my degree without commuting to Sul Ross State Teacher's College three hours away in a town with the unlikely name of Alpine, or leaving town for stretches unacceptable for a mother of young children.

I eagerly called for a course catalogue and went to register for the fall semester. I signed up for twenty-four credit hours. Shortly, the dean called me to his office to tell me this was impossible; nobody could do it. I assured him I could. We argued a while, and finally I promised to drop a course early in the semester if it seemed that the load was too heavy. This man obviously didn't understand how driven I was, how hungry to learn, and how motivated to get the paper that would confirm I had learned. I was a woman on a mission. And I knew that after my job at Head Start, school would be so easy.

It wasn't all that easy—UTPB had signed on some top-notch professors to come to this godforsaken campus, and they were determined to disprove the notion that West Texas had to be an intellectual wasteland. But it was fun. I loved to learn. I already had learned so much about child development and teaching by doing and by seeking out the knowledge from books and other sources. That made many of my courses a breeze. But I also liked to be challenged, so I immersed myself in sociology, social psychology, and communications courses that by now I knew were subjects I could devour for lunch every day and of which I would never tire.

At the end of the first semester, with twenty-four hours and all A's under my belt, I was called back to the dean's office and he apologized. That's how I managed to finish two years in one calendar year and graduate at the end of the summer of 1974 with more hours than I needed for a double major in speech communications and sociology, and all the classroom hours I needed to go for both elementary and secondary teaching certificates. I never did my student teaching, though, because it seems I was destined to take up the cause of reproductive rights.

As I made this journey, the women's movement helped me articulate my inchoate feeling that there was a good deal of basic unfairness about the narrow roles society assigned to me, and I became increasingly determined to do something about it.

Much of my volunteer work involved lending what support I could to the civil rights movement. In college I studied racial prejudice and the resultant injustices. I realized that women were being denied many fundamental rights, too, but this just wasn't noticed or discussed. For women to have full civil rights, we must have reproductive rights. Because if you can't manage your own fertility as you see fit, it is almost impossible to control anything else in your life.

 How my life would have changed for the worse, I believe, if the abortion option had not been readily available. Everything would have been different. I'm almost certain I would have struggled to go to college and most certainly wouldn't have moved to New York and worked on Wall Street. I know, that sounds selfish but I believe that young women in particular must be focused on their future as they enter the adult world. Lots of people (bosses who want secretaries and young men who want pretty faces rearing their children) have designs on them. In this case a little selfishness goes a long way. Some might say abortion takes lives. I would say it saves lives . . .

—Mercy, age forty

Always precocious, I had my midlife crisis at thirty-two. By this time, I knew I could not stay in my marriage, even if I lost all my friends and my family didn't love me any more. It had become impossible for me to live in someone else's skin. The integrity of my own being was paramount. I think you sometimes have to reach the bottom emotionally to start on your way up. It was a desperate feeling that the entire framework I had so carefully constructed to make myself the ideal wife of the 1950s and supermom of the '60s had collapsed. By then, our marriage had little substance and mainly the children in common. We were so young when we started out together that we had both grown into people who never would have married had we met at this point in our lives.

The children, who had been the center of my universe for so long, were teenagers. They increasingly had their own lives and weren't interested in mine—or so it seemed until we told them we were getting divorced. Then I realized how hard it had been for them to go through my metamorphosis from jelly woman to my very own handsome princess.

As my oldest, Tammy, then seventeen, exclaimed tearfully: "I just wish you had decided what you wanted to be before it would affect us so much. It wouldn't have been so bad if you had always been who you are now and we didn't have to go through the changes. We always had the perfect family. Now we don't." Ouch, knife to the already bleeding heart, no less painful for its ring of truth.

My friend Nona drew a picture of a butterfly emerging from its cocoon for my birthday, with the caption: "After you spread your wings, it's time for butterfly days." I still have it.

Chapter Six

This month's bills or this month's pills

 On September 11th, 2001, my mother, Valerie Joan Hanna, Senior Vice President, Technology at Marsh and McLennan was killed on the ninety-seventh floor of Tower One. She was a women's rights activist, who started as a single mom with two of her own, one adopted and somewhere around seventeen foster children over the years.

She worked her way up the corporate ladder, a key punch operator, hitting glass ceiling after glass ceiling, changing jobs often, moving on to companies with a higher glass ceiling ending up a Vice President on Wall Street of one of the largest multinational insurance firms.

We started with government cheese but even as she earned more money, rather than living the "good life" she helped more people and children get out of poverty. She provided each of us with an education to each of our individual abilities.

She was a very staunch reproductive rights supporter. Thank you for the work you do.

—In peace, Lydia J. Robertson

Lydia told me that what this American hero knew, and passed on to her children, is that poverty and too much pregnancy are as inextricably linked as the ability to control one's fertility and economic well-being.

The priest who introduced me to Planned Parenthood

For five years, in the 1960s and early '70s, I taught in the Odessa, Texas, Head Start program. I started out as a volunteer teacher's aide one day a week, and quickly became enthralled with early childhood education and obsessed with learning about every stage my own children were going through. I read every book on child development that I could get my hands on and my children became the victims of my desire to practice these new skills. The program was named Greater Opportunities of the Permian Basin, in keeping with the optimism of the era, as we set about lifting the economic status of all Americans, thereby eradicating many other injustices. Fittingly, the same War on Poverty also tiptoed gingerly into providing the first federal funding for family planning.

Volunteering at Head Start, especially in those heady days when it was a new program and not yet institutionalized as part of the public schools, was also a way for me to make a contribution to the civil rights movement. I felt passionately about it, but as a mother of preschoolers I couldn't go running off to Birmingham to march. So I did my part at home in West Texas.

The disparate threads of my life were beginning to weave themselves together as I gradually awakened to what was happening in the world around me, and connected the social issues of the day to myself and my family. West Texas wasn't exactly a hotbed of social change. I folded diapers while watching the nightly news and mentally, at least, traveled beyond Odessa thanks to the fascinating people who came into my living room via Jack Paar's *Tonight Show* long after the children were asleep.

My engagement in the civil rights movement had contributed to my transition from jelly woman to handsome princess. It toughened me up, emotionally and intellectually. I learned confrontation, and practiced speaking up and standing my ground when challenged. Those weren't things I'd learned growing up, but the underlying values of justice, fairness, and helping others were very much a part of my family. And, as I discovered once I began to study it—at about the same time—an integral part of Judaism, the heritage from which I'd distanced myself as a teenager in order not to be "different."

At first, I used those skills to help others. I've always found it easier to fight for someone else's rights than my own. Perhaps this is another jelly woman phenomenon, a feeling of unworthiness; perhaps it afflicts every minority that has a history of being oppressed. It was easier by far for me to confront racial and economic discrimination against African-Americans and Latinos than the anti-Semitism and sexism that affected me personally. Consciously or not, the civil rights movement sensitized me to the plight of others and in so doing taught me how to stand up for myself. But that would come later.

The woman who founded and ran Greater Opportunities was a crusty, crotchety, dyed-in-the-wool liberal (yes, even in West Texas, there were some) political junkie and journalist named Mildred Chaffin. In her own crusty, crotchety way, she became a mentor, often seeing in me abilities I did not see in myself.

After a year as a volunteer, I told her that I would not be able to continue because I had to get a paying job in the fall when my youngest entered kindergarten. She promptly offered me a teaching job even though my formal qualifications were limited. A few years later, she tapped me to develop a new concept, a parent-child communication program that recognized that children would be more successful in school if their parents participated in learning activities with them.

Mildred was a large white woman with bleached blonde hair. She was probably better suited by temperament to journalism than management, but she had a great and kind heart. She loved those children, though I doubt she could have stood up to one full day in the classroom. Once when she had officials visiting from Washington, she brought them around to my class. She was especially imposing that day in a white pique dress with red and blue costume jewelry. One little boy, who had obviously learned his lesson in rhyming, piped up, "Red, white and blue, the monkey favors you," mortifying both of us and giving the officials a good laugh.

My class was held in the parish hall of the Catholic Church in the poorest part of town. The priest once said to me, "How can I tell these people to have a baby every year? I can't feed them. I can't take care of all of them." I had no idea how radical this was for a Catholic priest to say, but I certainly knew his compassionate words made sense to me. I've often wondered how he fared in the priesthood later on.

Poverty and pregnancy and pregnancy and poverty

The other teacher in that parish hall and a leading lay member of the church agreed with him, and she took the moms of the children in her class to Planned Parenthood every month for their birth control supplies. This overlap between the two programs, and the people who supported them, was repeated around the country. The connections between poverty and the lack of knowledge about family planning and access to services were made manifest in so many ways.

Yes, the families we served were all poor. But I could so clearly see the differences among them. The children from small families generally were more alert, better clothed and fed, and had more positive attitudes. Their parents were the ones who had the time and resources to participate in my new parent-child communications program. While it wasn't by any means a perfect correlation, I observed that when we held our daily "magic circles"—where we discussed feelings and practiced social skills—the children from the most impoverished homes either had great difficulty learning to control their aggression or they had become so passive they had difficulty interacting at all.

This is not meant to disparage large families where resources are adequate to care for the children. I could write a book about the joys of being with my own family of eight cousins. But I could see, very concretely, every day in my classroom, how family planning had helped children by allowing their parents to improve their own lives. I certainly knew from my own experience that reliable birth control had given me my health, my sanity, and the ability to seek the education that qualified me for employment. I thought it only fair that other women and families have the same chance to pull themselves up as I'd had.

Everything I've learned since validates my early observations about the benefits of thoughtfully planned families and spaced pregnancies. Mothers, children, families, and society all benefit.

Curing the epidemic lack of health care access

Women today talk about the value of family planning and reproductive health care in their own lives:

 Without this institution, I would not have medical care for gynecological visits. My insurance company doesn't cover Pap smears and pelvic exams unless you are pregnant. Now I can prevent pregnancy until I am ready to start my family.

—Jane, age twenty-two

 I have very little insurance coverage and am still a student. If I can't afford insurance, I could hardly afford to support a child.

—Rose, age twenty-five

As our nation faces hunger, child abuse, homelessness and rising domestic violence, it is hard for me to imagine how our federal, state and local governments can possibly consider, not to mention actually cut the budget for the very people it is supposed to help. Welfare cuts are one thing but when a woman's health and choice to not reproduce is violated it should be a crime. It has become an epidemic in this nation that so many are without insurance. As the saying goes, "An ounce of prevention is worth a pound of cure."

We have three children that we love very much, but we choose to not have more. Family planning is important. I don't want my tubes tied but I do need choices.

Family planning helps me care for my body so I can care for my family. If I can't do this the burden may be shifted back to the state by way of food stamps, Medicaid, etc.

My ounce of prevention lies in family planning so the pound of cure won't be on the state.

—Eve, thirties

 I had lost my job with no health care and having pain in my abdomen. Without subsidized clinics the cyst in my ovaries would have gone unnoticed and untreated. Going to a regular doctor is way too expensive.

—Molly, age twenty-seven

 I was seventeen when I had my son Jack. I made a mistake but at least can go to a clinic that helps me prevent making the same mistake. I can't afford $27 a month for birth control pills. I can't pay for my annual Pap smears that tell me I am healthy and cancer free. I haven't found another place where I have someone to talk to about sex and how to be responsible, what kind of birth control is best for me.

—Annie, age twenty-one

There are so many women who regularly have to choose between this month's bills and this month's pills. Millions live in the gray area between government subsidized health care and employer-provided insurance. Author Barbara Ehrenreich lived among them for months as she wrote *Nickel and Dimed: On (Not) Getting by in America*. She talks about Maddy, a single mom who cleans houses but has to stretch to find the $50 she pays for child care, and Holly, also a maid, trying to work amid the harsh chemicals in spite of overwhelming pregnancy-related nausea. Writes Ehrenreich, "But the relevant point about Holly is that she is visibly unwell—possibly whiter, on a daily basis, than anyone else in the state. We're not just talking Caucasian here; think bridal gowns, tuberculosis, and death. All I know about her is that she is twenty-three, has been married for almost a year, and manages to feed her husband, herself, and an elderly relative on $30-50 a week."

Worldwide, women comprise 70 percent of those who live in poverty—a condition created by their low status in the family and in society. They have less access to education and therefore less ability to earn a living. Throw into the mix lack of control over fertility, and the situation is exacerbated. There's no way out of poverty for a woman whose health and income are compromised by her inability to stop becoming pregnant.

Recent research has identified the challenges women face when trying to move out of poverty. According to the Manpower Demonstration Research Corporation, women on welfare and unemployed women have significantly more health problems than their better-off counterparts. And the kinds of problems that the researchers found—depression, children who are less healthy than the norm, homelessness, obesity—made it difficult for them to work.

The societal costs are as high as the personal ones—low birth weight babies, welfare dependency, the impact of unwantedness on the crime rate, unintended pregnancy and its subsequent costs, and much more. In the U.S., study after study shows that every public dollar spent on family planning returns three dollars in avoided government-funded health care costs in just the very first year.

Global voices

In the developing world, the largest childbearing generation in history—over one billion young people between fifteen and twenty-four—is in its prime reproductive years. In addition, 150 million married women would limit their family size or space their families if they had access to contraception. Throughout the world, 350 million

couples are not able to get the family planning services and contraceptives they want.

In the words of Rohsana Kahondokar, a lawyer in Bangladesh, where
contraceptive use rose from 3 percent of the population to 60 percent
of the population in twenty-five years:

> Family planning leads to economy planning leads to national
> planning. And central to it all is the changing role of women.
> After all, a country cannot develop with the participation of
> only half its citizens.

The next story offers a glimpse of the human suffering that's behind those numbers. The writer calls it, "How I became a family plan-
ner at age eleven."

> I grew up on the Mexico border in Arizona, where women
> were willing to cross the border to work for $3 a day. My mother
> later joked that it was thanks to Juana that she could never be
> attorney general of the U.S. Juana worked for us one day a
> week for most of my childhood. Every year, she took a vaca-
> tion in the fall. From what we could understand with our lim-
> ited Spanish, she traveled to Mexico City to visit her husband,
> who worked there. A few months after she returned, we could
> see she was pregnant. The inevitable finally happened. She didn't
> show up for work and we heard that the baby was stillborn.
> And that she didn't have the money to pay the tax required
> before burial.
>
> All the people she worked for contributed money, food,
> clothes and more to help her and her family. My father was
> charged with delivering it all—he had driven her all of the way
> home several times, when it was raining, instead of just leaving
> her at the border. He was the only one who knew where she
> lived. I was about eleven. I went with him as he drove through

streets the likes of which I had never seen; essentially, rutted, dirt paths. We passed the community well where women were doing laundry and filling water jugs. We were only a few miles from my three-bedroom, two-bath house with air conditioning and a dishwasher. My three sisters and I complained about sharing bedrooms. Juana's house was one small room with adobe walls and a dirt floor. There was an icebox (without any ice) in the corner and a table in the middle of the room. On the table, covered with oilcloth, was the body of the baby boy.

We gave her the money and the goods and, without changing her stoic facial expression, she cried. Her children sat silently on the floor. My father told her not to worry about work; she could come back when she was ready. She assured him that her oldest daughter would work in her place until she came back. Sure enough, when Mom drove to the border to pick her up, Juana's daughter was ready for work. She was only a few years older than I was. And she was pregnant.

—Carol, age forty-six

It may be difficult for those of us who have not been in such a situation to understand the despair that can accompany poverty. Even with a steady income, I remember what it was like to have three small children and not an extra dollar to spend. We were lucky—one set of parents had a farm and one had a clothing factory, so we always had meat, fresh fruit and vegetables, and fabric to make clothes. Talk about Suzy Homemaker—I canned and froze, jellied and preserved, and sewed like I knew what I was doing. My oldest daughter, Tammy, once remarked that we had everything her more affluent friends had— we just didn't have as much space to put it in. The habits became ingrained even though my circumstances are different now. To this day, I rarely buy a cup of fancy coffee on the way to the office like I see so many people doing, and it really annoys me when they try to sell you bottled water in a restaurant. And I wouldn't dream of throwing away those little sliver ends of soap; they must be smooshed onto the next bar.

Fertility control equals life control

I remember the panic and desperation that accompanied the threat of pregnancy when my mental, physical, and emotional resources were stretched to the breaking point by three small children—and the great relief that the birth control pill brought into my life. So I could empathize, years later, when our director of clinics came to my management staff to ask for help. She needed contributions to pay for an abortion for an impoverished woman with four children who, when she discovered she was pregnant again, climbed onto the roof of her trailer and tried to throw herself off.

Fertility control is the key to improving a woman's mental and physical health and her economic status, and when that care is not affordable, she has to make heart-rending choices. But if a woman can control her fertility, she has a chance to control other parts of her life. When the light goes on for women in those situations as it did for me, here's what they say:

 The divorce has impoverished me, going back to school is so expensive but it is my only way out of this. I was married for twenty-five years and then he divorced me. I live with my parents, work full time and all the money goes out to pay off bills, or for school. I really don't know what I would do without low-cost care. I won't be poor forever then maybe I can help someone else.

—Joanne, age forty-four

 I'm a single parent with four children. I myself didn't finish school, I drop out at the age fifteen to start a family. After paying rent light and the other utilities, there's not enough to support myself or my children. This is why I'm asking for a loan to pay for my daughter's abortion. Because I myself know that she will not finish school. Please help me and my daughter in this horrible cycle that needs to be broken. She's in school and I want her to finish so she can see a better future than what I have. I know the cycle can be broken because I have a son who is eighteen years old. And he is graduating this following next year. And he has no children at all.

—Connie, age thirty-four

 Being able to plan a family allows a woman independence, especially low-income women like myself. A lot of us who use the low-cost services are struggling to get off welfare and striving for independence. I myself have been off welfare for a year now. I have been able to hold a job for the past four years, accumulated money in the bank, live in a house I renovated myself and plan to go to college next year. For myself, unplanned pregnancy would be a major setback in my goals to make a better life.

—Elna, age twenty-eight

To be poor even in the richest country on earth means subordinating your sexuality and even your health to the more pressing needs of food and shelter. But subsidized family planning services can turn sob stories into success stories, as they did for Dallas City Council Representative Veletta Forsythe Lill:

 Planned Parenthood possibly saved my life. Eighteen years ago, my husband decided to quit his very lucrative corporate job and pursue his dream of being an airline pilot. He needed, as they say in the trade, to "build hours," so he accepted a position with a commuter airline. And, so, we struggled for several years while he built his hours and we put off a lot of priorities. For me, one of those was annual exams. And I went several years without having an annual exam. I finally decided it was time and we still didn't have a lot of money and I chose, knowing that Planned Parenthood has services that I could access for a low cost, I chose to go to the Planned Parenthood organization in my city. To make a long story short, I had an irregular Pap smear—a surgical procedure. My husband built his hours—he is now a captain of American Airlines, we are the proud parents of a twelve-year- old boy, and we all lived happily ever after. I want to thank you for giving me a past and a future.

Other women describe their circumstances in plain terms:

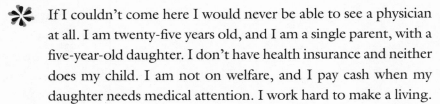 If I couldn't come here I would never be able to see a physician at all. I am twenty-five years old, and I am a single parent, with a five-year-old daughter. I don't have health insurance and neither does my child. I am not on welfare, and I pay cash when my daughter needs medical attention. I work hard to make a living.

—Nancy, age twenty-five

My Mother's Day present this year was and is the best I've had in a while. My daughter got me a free Pap test . . . She knew it had been years since I had one. My family's history is riddled with cancer. We don't have health insurance because it's not affordable.

—Leola, age forty-five

Since the birth of my daughter in 1995 I've used [subsidized] services. Being a working single mother my profession as a cosmetologist doesn't provide health insurance. My income varies weekly. So thanks to the help and income support of the clinic I am able to stay healthy. I'm not an unwed mother bringing children into this world that I cannot support. Would you rather lower our birth rates or fund welfare families? Keep America's women healthy.

—Tiffany, age twenty-five

 I am a twenty-one-year-old mother of three children. I was under a lot of stress for the fact that I have no health insurance to cover me. Medi-Cal will not cover me because me and my husband make too much money, but we don't make enough to buy a private insurance plan. This clinic has been the greatest miracle that I have come across.

—Sabrina, age twenty-one

Absence of hope

Many of the women who write are so young, or were teen mothers just as I was. Having children too young contributes to their poverty and dependency; poverty and dependency contribute to high rates of unintended and teen pregnancies. Esperanza Garcia Walters, a social worker who works with high-risk, low-income teens, tells this story about the effects of poverty on teen girls and why avoiding pregnancy isn't necessarily a priority for them:

 I asked a group of teen mothers to share their dreams and aspirations with me. I was disheartened to discover that they really didn't see much of a future for themselves. Later, it hit me. It wasn't that these girls had no dreams; it was that they had no hope.

Esperanza then compared these girls to others in the same situation who had the advantage of participating in a program that taught them about options and social skills, with a healthy dose of sexuality and family planning education thrown in. She said the program gave the young women the hope they needed to become motivated to delay further childbearing and pursue their dreams.

Once, when I was in Arizona, a woman with three little children in tow came to our Prescott clinic for a pregnancy test. She lived way out in the country and getting into town wasn't easy for her. Her husband had just left her—and he had left her with a raging sexually transmitted infection. She knew she needed help. She brought with her a dozen eggs and a carton of milk. She announced that she had just spent the last of her last money on these items for her children. She did not know how she would pay for the medical care she so desperately needed.

President Bush as advocate for family planning?
No, not that George Bush.

What the woman with the eggs and milk didn't know was that we had funding to cover her services from a program called Title X of the Public Health Services Act. One of its original sponsors, a Midland, Texas, oilman, Congressman George H.W. Bush, said, "We need to make family planning a household word. We need to take the sensationalism out of the topic so it can no longer be used by militants who have no knowledge of the voluntary nature of the program, but rather are using it as a political stepping stone."

This was 1970, of course—before he sold his pro-choice principles to become Ronald Reagan's vice president. Bush went on to say—at least in 1970—"If family planning is anything, it is a public health matter."

A public health matter indeed.

Fortunately for our patient, Title X paid for her services, she wasn't pregnant, and her infection was treatable. She continued as a patient at the clinic, and the staff told me later that she was able to get a job in town. Her story illustrates exactly why access to reproductive health services is the key to giving women a chance to succeed in life.

I fear for what may happen to women like her in the future, now that President George W. Bush and many Congressmen want to shift family planning funding to useless abstinence-only sex-ed programs, that is if they can't kill family planning programs and defund them entirely. All those sanctimonious politicians who try to use women's reproductive health and rights as political stepping stones, should listen to this twenty-eight-year-old woman, who says it best:

 Times are hard and children are expensive.

Chapter Seven

Making family

The birds and the bees and the Petri dish

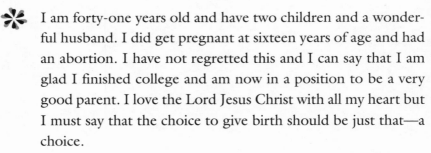 I am forty-one years old and have two children and a wonderful husband. I did get pregnant at sixteen years of age and had an abortion. I have not regretted this and I can say that I am glad I finished college and am now in a position to be a very good parent. I love the Lord Jesus Christ with all my heart but I must say that the choice to give birth should be just that—a choice.

—Lucy, age forty-one

They are years of excruciating agony and limitless joy. Years in which we make the decisions—or fall into the situations—that define the course of our lives. Years when our families are shaped, our careers are launched, our worlds are created.

Who controls the power to create life?

Consider the years when women's unique power, the power to create life, comes to fruition—or doesn't, by choice, or by fluke of

96

nature. Years when (in eras past—and even today, in some places and in some minds) fear or envy or resentment of that awesome power led to the inequality and injustices that ensured women had no other power. Yes, even today, when the debate supposedly is about "life," and "choice," it is really about who has the control over a woman's power to create life. I spent those years in the sheltered world of Odessa, Texas, where my three children grew up surrounded by families that, at least on the surface, looked a lot like us, where we were all trying to look like *Father Knows Best*.

At the time the light bulb—that I might someday have to support these children in that wider world beyond my circumscribed life — went off in my head (shortly after my son, David, was born, and he still refers to himself as "Mom's light bulb") I was barely twenty. Two method failures and one episode of magical thinking and, bingo, I had three children. At one every other year, I could end up with fifteen more pregnancies before nature mercifully took me out of commission. I had severe anemia with my last two pregnancies, and I was so exhausted that I was losing weight involuntarily for the first and only time in my life. The Pill had reached Odessa, Texas, by then and I started popping those high-hormone Enovid E's like they were candy. The hell with the side effects. I knew that having another child right then would send me over the brink, physically and emotionally.

At least I had the option of the Pill. Consider this letter from Margaret Sanger's 1928 book, *Motherhood in Bondage:*

 I am the mother of five children, four living . . . and I had one miscarriage. I have had to work six years at night to support my children as I have a husband who drinks and does not care if we live or not. Every month I'm in dread of being pregnant I have only a year and eight months between two of my children and I think I would rather die than ever have any more. Not that I don't love them but it is so hard.

And then from the perspective of a child born during that era, to a mother without choices, activist Linn Duvall Harwell told me why she has dedicated her life to reproductive rights in order to improve the lives of women everywhere:

 I was born into an overpopulated house in an ethnic neighborhood in Pittsburgh. I was thrust into the population field shortly after my sixth birthday by the death of my thirty-four year-old mother from a self-inflicted abortion. Our family was so damaged as to stunt our intellectual and social growth. Each of the siblings suffered in individual ways. At sixteen, when I learned why my mother died, I determined this would not happen to me.

Linn was able to get contraception when she married at nineteen in 1942. She and she husband planned their four children, and just celebrated their sixtieth anniversary.

The power of the Pill

Birth control—at least the desire to control fertility, if not always the means—has been around forever. As early as 1850 B.C., evidence suggests that vaginal suppositories concocted from crocodile dung and honey were used to try to prevent pregnancies, whether or not what caused them was truly understood. Until recent times, methods were rudimentary and less than optimally effective. A Texas woman in her seventies remembers her own mother's idea of birth control—an easily obtainable but not always effective method still practiced in many parts of the world today:

 Mama had a trick, she kept breastfeeding my youngest sister until that baby was three years old because she thought that would keep her from getting pregnant. She already had seven children, and one dead. We lived on a farm, and it was hard work. By and by, she quit breastfeeding. And boom, she was pregnant.

Thanks to the Pill and other modern means of birth control, women have moved from trying to stop having children after three or five or ten—like these two women did, and like I did decades later—to planning even a very first pregnancy and spacing subsequent births, like my own children have done. Making family has moved from making the best of the whims of nature to making the best decisions for your family.

The only thing that hasn't changed is that nothing touches our humanity, our souls, more than when it touches our family. Here are just a few variations on that theme:

 Ignorance infuriates me. My husband and I are married fifty years this month. We never had much money; we're both Catholics and don't believe in the theory that 'the more the better.' (It just ain't true.) Had we continued to create babies, ours and their lives would not have been good ones. Quality not quantity is important. It takes a toll on a woman's body as well. Some of us are simply not strong enough to carry baby after baby for nine months. We had three babies: two sons and one daughter. They have grown into beautiful adults with successful lives and parents who love them and were able to care for them properly in very small quarters.

—Peggy, age seventy-three

 I was sixteen years old with the man who became my husband. He was first person I slept with and was not very knowledgeable about birth control. I knew what was out there, but did not know how to reach it. I had had an appointment to begin taking birth control pills when I missed a period. I took a urine test and found out I was pregnant. Everyone in the office was very helpful and told me what my options were. I knew being a sophomore in high school I could not have that baby. They were very helpful and helped me with all the steps to an abortion. I have always been pro-life, but you cannot say what you would do unless you were in the situation. I do not regret what I did. I am in college now pursuing my teaching career and I know I did what was right for me. I am very fond of children and hope to have some when I am ready . . . but for now I am using birth control pills *and* condoms until I am ready for them.

—Alana, age twenty-three

In 1986 I received low-cost ob-gyn care and birth control. I had no insurance and felt uncomfortable asking my parents to help me in this manner. Because I was able to receive practically free birth control pills, I never had to deal with an unplanned pregnancy and was therefore able to finish college and plan and pursue a career. Now, as an older, married professional, I can plan a family that I am ready for, financially and emotionally.

—Beatrice, age thirty-four

I was thirty-four, engaged to a wonderful man, pregnant, and my fiancé and our families were very excited! Because of my age, my doctor encouraged me to undergo amniocentesis. To our dismay, the baby tested positive for Down's syndrome, and other related birth defects. We made the sad choice of abortion. I know that it was the right thing to do, as I could not handle a child with potentially serious birth defects. The procedure went without a hitch, by the most wonderful Dr. Slepian, and I have no regrets about my decision. I will always fight to keep abortion safe and legal and have vowed to do my part to keep the clinics accessible.

—Nancy, age forty-four

On October 23, 1998, Dr. Barnett Slepian was assassinated in the kitchen of his home while his children watched. The alleged murderer is a "pro-life" domestic terrorist currently waiting to be tried.

Birth control and legal abortion gave these women, and me, so much more than fertility control. It is not an overstatement—it's a jubilant statement of fact—to say that fertility control gives women nothing short of control over their lives. That joy permeates the stories like the ones above, many of them from women who cherish the family, the career, the strong marriage that they now have and therefore deeply value the role that birth control and abortion played in their ability to achieve all those dreams. Nearly half of all women in the U.S. have had an abortion by the time they are forty-five years old. Abortion, too, is a part of making family—of having all options available at all times to all people.

How could I, for example, have managed to go to school, to reclaim the intellect that I'd abandoned at fifteen, when I already was physically exhausted, with three small children to care for, and the threat of another pregnancy hanging over my head? As it was, it took me twelve years to finish my degree. Although I always knew, on some level, that I'd go back to school—I had absorbed those Jewish values of social responsibility and education through my pores—when I did, I still operated on another level, always the wife and mother first, never letting school interfere with dinner on the table and clean clothes in the closet.

Fifties fallacies

That's what the world looked like in the late 1950s and early '60s in Odessa, Texas. Rosie the Riveter had been put back in her place as Suzy Homemaker. Post-war government subsidies of education and home ownership had created large pockets of suburban sanctuary. My children ran in and out of our house and the neighbors' houses all day long, and came home at night to the house Aunt Ida's bequest of $500 in U.S. savings bonds had helped us buy. But not far away, African-Americans, Latinos, and other minorities almost uniformly were left out of this prosperity thanks to segregation, discriminatory real estate policies, harassment, violence, and other ugly reminders of an America that had yet to extend the American dream to all its citizens.

The roles of both women and men were strictly defined, and the societal pressure to conform was fierce. According to Stephanie Coontz in *The Way We Never Were,* women "who had trouble adjusting to 'creative homemaking,' were labeled neurotic, perverted, or schizophrenic. . . . Men were also pressured into acceptable family roles, since lack of a suitable wife could mean the loss of a job or promotion." Rather than a time of traditional values (whatever they are), it was a time of the highest teenage pregnancy rates we've ever seen. As Coontz says, "Young people were not taught how to 'say no'—they were simply handed wedding rings."

Beneath the surface, Ozzie didn't have a clue, Harriett was becoming Betty Friedan (or wishing she was Marlo Thomas), and the kids were wondering why everyone else on the street had a perfect family.

Coontz says, "[G]rowing up in the 1950s . . . was not so much a matter of being protected from the harsh realities of the outside world as preventing the outside world from learning the harsh realities of family life. Few would have guessed that radiant Marilyn Van Derbur, crowned Miss America in 1958, had been sexually violated by her wealthy, respectable father from the time she was five. By 1960, almost every major news journal was using the word trapped to describe the feelings of the American housewife."

I can't imagine, for the life of me, why anyone would be nostalgic for such a world, for such unrealistic, unjust views of what family should be. The truth is that family has always been what we make it—defined not by some politician's blueprint or a hazy, romanticized dream of what it never was but by each family's unique fingerprint.

Sixties ironies

When the day came that I couldn't take the Pill anymore, the gynecologist and obstetrician who delivered two of my children made arrangements for me to go to Ector County Hospital to have a laproscopic tubal sterilization—a new procedure then. I went alone because my husband had to stay home to get the kids off to school and then he had to go off to work or lose a day's pay. The woman who signed me in told me that I would have to get his signature. That made my new feminist hackles rise, and I told her that that was impossible but mainly that it was unfair—I was the one who got pregnant, after all. When it became clear that I wasn't going to budge, she called my doctor, probably assuming that he would decline my request. Dr. Keith Oehlschlager calmed her down and pretty soon, she turned back to me and handed me the consent form with nary a word.

That was my small victory, a victory for the family I cherished and wanted. It's no wonder that women throughout time have felt so strongly about whether and when to bear a child that history is filled with stories of the desperate measures they have taken to control their fertility. Even today, nearly half of all women in the U.S. who have had legal abortions say they would consider, or would definitely have, an illegal one—risking health and life—if that were their only choice. And the truth—if history is any predictor—is that almost all of them would.

Often the medical establishment has been both the problem and the solution. It fought to outlaw abortion late in the nineteenth century because midwives performed them, and that represented money not going into doctors' pockets. And it created one imperfect and patently unfair solution by providing relatively safe but illegal abortions to women with money.

 Forty-three years ago, I was twenty-eight and pregnant with my second child—first one, twenty-two months old. Crossing a main artery in my Volkswagen on a green light, a Buick went through his red light and hit my car—I was thrown out at eight-

and-one-half months. After delivery the next month, the OB told me not to get pregnant again. After my husband and I talked it over, I told my doctor our decision to have a tubal ligation. It was explained to me that it wasn't a law but the doctors in our state couldn't perform sterilization unless the mother's age times the number of children she had equaled one hundred and twenty—with my two, I would be eligible at 60. I asked what would happen if I did get pregnant . . . was told not to worry, they would perform a D&C . . . you know what that is (an abortion by another name). What irony.

—Betty, age seventy-one

I found out after I started working for Planned Parenthood that my personal physician, the remarkable Dr. "O," who allowed me to consent to my own surgery, was the volunteer medical director there. A devout Methodist who raised orchids in his greenhouse, he had been providing safe abortion in his private practice for years, even before *Roe v. Wade* made it legal. He told me that it was such a wonderful feeling to help so many women; they were so grateful.

Families valued

What a blessing it is to women that they can elect to delay child-bearing while pursuing other life goals, such as advanced education and careers, just as men have always been able to do—a key factor in the improvement of the status of women in the twentieth century. What a blessing to their children and their families that they can give birth when they are most able to raise a child.

 I decided that after three children I needed to go back to school. With my busy schedule I kept forgetting to take my pills. The Depo-Provera shot is great.

—Willa, age twenty-eight

Both times I decided that having my children was the best choice for me. About a year ago I found out that I was pregnant again and this time I knew that I couldn't handle another baby. I have a wonderful husband and a great job. I did indeed have an abortion and have thought of it often since but I know that it was the right decision for me and my family. I am glad I had that option.

—Anabel, age twenty-two

 When I found out I was pregnant with my first pregnancy it was a new territory for me. I was twenty years old, newly married and here I was expecting! What would the future bring with this baby on the way. I wasn't sure if we could financially afford this little one. I knew I had options. I choose the option that was the right choice for me! My future was brightened when I gave birth to a beautiful baby girl who is the treasure of my life. And three years later I gave birth to my second daughter! What a gift motherhood has been for me.

—Bridget, age twenty-nine

 I am a student in a college and I got pregnant the summer of my freshman year. With no money to my name and no one to help take care of the baby once it came, I opted for an abortion. It was hard for me to save up enough to pay for that but I knew that I did not want to bring a baby into the world that I could not take care of. There are already so many neglected children I didn't want to add to that population. I will one day begin again on a family, but I will be prepared. Until then I am abstaining from sex because I feel that I owe that to the child I gave up and the children I hope to have in the future. I have now met a wonderful guy who supports and cares for me, we are saving up now (as we are both still in college) to buy a house and start preparing to start a family. I know that I will never forget what course of action I took before and I will never be able to repay the clinic for the lifesaver . . . mine. Without it, I wouldn't be who I am today and I would have been unable to provide anything for my child.

—Courtney, age twenty

These are individual stories, but the ability to control fertility through contraception and abortion has broad implications for society as a whole, and for the health of women and children. The Centers for Disease Control and Prevention calls family planning one of the ten most important medical advances of the twentieth century. The anthropologist and social philosopher Ashley Montagu says the Pill is as important as the discovery of fire and the invention of tools.

Infant mortality has declined dramatically; the health of women has improved significantly; and families are strengthened. Unwanted children are more likely to have chaotic and insecure family lives, perform more poorly in school, exhibit delinquent behavior, and require psychiatric treatment. One study credits legal abortion for half of the drop in the crime rate in the 1990s. Although the study has been criticized, predictably, by anti-choice forces, common sense suggests that women who give birth to wanted children are likely to be more nurturing, with predictable results.

 When I was a teenager in Alabama I had a friend whose family did foster care for infants. They often took in babies who were underweight and addicted to crack, or whose mental and physical disabilities caused their parents to give them up. These babies were shuttled from foster home to foster home, unwanted and unhealthy. Abortions and birth control are very difficult to find in the South. If more women had access to these services there would be fewer children born addicted, born in poverty, living in abusive homes, and born to parents who don't want them.

—Candice, age forty-one

Dr. Martin Luther King Jr., in a May 1966 speech, agreed: "There is scarcely anything more tragic in human life than a child who is not wanted. That which should be a blessing becomes a curse for parent and child."

 I used to be against abortion. My theory was: You made your bed, now lie in it. Then I realized that it was the parents who should have to suffer the consequences. Why should the child? There's adoption but how many babies are adopted? Most of them will end up in the system (have you heard the horror stories that foster kids go through) and repeat the process over again. So I'm pro choice because sometimes there is no other option. Even for those who aren't I don't think they should judge, not until they have to make a choice as difficult as this one.

—Hannah, age thirty-nine

 If individuals are not informed, there would be many more unwanted pregnancies resulting in uncared for children. I do not think a child should pay–by being mistreated–for its parents' mistakes.

—Charles, age twenty-six

Technology and social values

To women, families, children, and to me, easy-to-use, effective birth control was a personal miracle. But the Pill popped into a society that was in the midst of great change—the civil rights movement, the push for equal rights for women, and more. That pill was both a catalyst for change and a target for those who feared that change. And like most world-changing new technologies, it leaped ahead of social values.

From Reverend Stephen J. Mather, a Presbyterian minister in Anaheim, California:

The Pill is a fundamental problem to established authority. It allows a woman to independently, if she wishes, make her own decision about her own life. The Pill is the place where religion, sex and politics all come out of the closet. It forced us to discuss the nature of sex—was it only for reproduction?—and the nature of power—who has it, who doesn't?

The chemist Carl Djerassi, whose synthesis of a female hormone from a wild Mexican yam made the Pill's development possible, reflecting on the uproar that ensued from his discovery:

 I am convinced that if we had synthesized norethindrone (later) than 1951 . . . oral contraceptives would not have existed in the year 2000 . . . because hardly any pharmaceutical company with the financial, logistic and marketing muscle necessary to bring oral contraceptives to the market (because of clinical trial restrictions and litigation fears) would have been willing to carry on during the 1980s and 1990s.

He's right. The fight to introduce mifepristone (early nonsurgical abortion) in the U.S. is a case in point. It's only been available here for early, medical abortion since September 2000, in spite of the fact that women in Europe have had access to it for more than ten years. Politics and fallout from social change, not medical caution, kept mifepristone out of the U.S.

Mother Nature's mean streak

A friend of mine says she knows God is male because of the way the female reproductive system is designed to provide far more fertility than most families would ever want and with such high degree of bother and muss. If we didn't already believe it, a look at reproductive capability would be enough to prove that life isn't fair. We get pregnant when we don't want to, then can't when we want to. Mother Nature either has a wicked sense of humor or a mean streak.

The number of couples with infertility problems is growing. People are marrying later, and therefore trying to start families after their fertility has begun to decline. And greater numbers of people today have fertility problems related to sexually transmitted infections. Technology has responded, bringing as it usually does exciting new choices along with troubling moral dilemmas. There are so many options that a recent public television broadcast of *Nova* started with the premise that there were eighteen different ways to make a baby and then found many more. Birth control, legal abortion, new reproductive technologies, and rapid social change have given us a much more complex world than the one Margaret Sanger faced.

 I am thirty-three and have been married for nearly ten years. I found out four years ago that I can't have children, and there's nothing more that can be done to help me medically. My experience with infertility and infertility treatment have made me even more convinced that every reproductive choice is so intensely personal that the state simply cannot rightly interfere. When I started exploring adoption, others again started asking if I hadn't changed my pro-choice belief. I haven't. I hope someday I will find a child to parent. But I also hope that child will come to me as a result of another woman's choice, freely made, and not because she has no other option available to her.

—Jill, age thirty-three

 When my husband and I made the decision to become parents, we did so joyfully and after much thought. It felt strange when, for the first time, I left the diaphragm in its case and had sex with the intention to procreate. It felt even stranger when pregnancy—the result I had so carefully avoided for nearly a decade—did not occur immediately. Months ran into years, and we gradually realized we had an infertility problem. Years of tests and medical procedures followed. My reproductive abilities, so long an intensely private and self-controlled function of my womanhood, became an almost public topic, dictated by forces out of my control and studied by dozens of students at the teaching hospital where we sought infertility treatment.

As a long-time pro-choice advocate, I was surprised when many of my friends and acquaintances expected my views about reproductive choice to change when we faced infertility. Quite the opposite. As my choices vanished with each failed medical procedure or unavailable option, I became even more convinced that ideally, women and men should make these decisions privately, without outside intervention unless it is specifically sought.

When we resolved our infertility through adoption, we faced new challenges. Most of the private adoption agencies we contacted were faith-based, and many of them required us to attest—sometimes with a witness such as our minister—that we were morally opposed to abortion. We could not make that pledge, not even in the context of our now almost desperate search for a baby. We found only one local adoption agency that didn't require such a promise, and through them we were joyfully matched with our son.

As we waited with the birth mother for the foster mother to bring the child, desperate to make small talk, we all began gingerly discussing our impressions of the 2000 election. We had a collective sigh of relief when it became obvious that we'd each voted for the same candidate. At the same time, however, I silently tensed—this particular election had, for me, come to down to a single issue: reproductive choice. I was not at all sure I wanted to engage in a discussion of abortion rights with my son's birth mother just moments before she was to place him into my arms forever.

And then an amazing thing happened. Our birth mother began speaking, quietly at first and then with more passion, about her strong belief in the right of each woman to make her own decisions about whether to carry a child to term. She told her own story and reminded us that she had chosen to give birth to—and then make an adoption plan for—her baby. Remarkably, she asked us to be sure to convey to our son, when he was old enough to understand, that she respected the rights of women who choose abortion just as much as she honored her own choice. She asked that we never allow him to view his own adoption as fuel for an anti-choice point of view. "Make sure he knows that," she asked. Today, he does know that. As he sees his mother continue to advocate for reproductive freedoms, he is aware of his birth mother's respect for each woman's individual choice.

—Lee Ann, thirties

Many ways of making family

Sometimes, it is not infertility but sexual orientation that leads to new technological and ethical issues. Increased options for childbearing have given gay men and lesbians the ability to assert their desire to make families.

 Devin's mom is a lesbian who had donor insemination to conceive him. My lover, Jim, and I are co-parents; Devin lives one week with her and one week with us. His mother decided when he was growing up she would be very open with him about his origins so he was very aware and the other kids in school knew. When he was in second or third grade, all the children were asked to do little scrapbook biographies. The first page of his autobiography was the cancelled check for the semen donation. So Devin is unusually empathetic. Around the same time he came home from school one day, and we were talking, and he said, "I don't understand, some of the kids at school seem so isolated and unhappy and there seem to be so many of them. How can that be?" I said, "Well, you know, Devin, not all families plan on having children." "What?" exclaimed this most carefully planned child. "Well, a lot of people have children by having sexual intercourse without thinking about having children so many children are born by accident." "Haven't they ever heard of condoms?" Devin said.

You see, he was raised with this sense that parenthood was something very volitional, that people decided carefully that they wanted to raise a child. He was shocked, he was really shocked, that something as important as having a child could be an accident.

Things are moving so fast that by the time he was in the fifth grade his teacher, a lesbian, and her life-partner had decided to have a child and (with the parents' involvement) came out to the kids about the pregnancy. One little girl asked if the father was a redhead but another little girl interrupted and said, "Don't be silly, he isn't the father. He's the donor. A father is someone who plays a role in your life. This is just about semen."

—Jon, age fifty-nine

Technology and changing times have stretched our thinking about what makes a family; indeed, the very definition of who is a parent is in serious legal and ethical flux. Is it the sperm donor? The woman who contributes the egg? How about the woman whose uterus houses the embryo? Or the parents who raise the child? All of the above?

The answers can be found in each story, for each one is the story of one family, of one choice, of one child, of his or her future. Each one underscores my contention that yesterday, today, tomorrow, in decades and centuries past, for years to come, and throughout all time, there is only one thing that can make a family: not laws, not speeches, not even blood. Only love can make a family.

Reverand Philip A. Wogaman of Foundry United Methodist Church in Washington, DC, affirmed that at a Planned Parenthood prayer breakfast:

 First, responsible parenting is a work of divine love. I do not think there is any human task more important than the procreation and nurturing of the young. Some people conclude from this that there should be as many new lives as possible, since there is no condition worse than the condition of never having been born. But God did not create us with limitless potential. If children are to be what God intends them to be, they must be surrounded by love and each given the opportunity to fulfill their potentialities. Real love for children means having the number of children that one can care for responsibly and lovingly. Some are not suited by temperament or age; sometimes external conditions are not yet right. Bringing every conceivable child into existence (the pun is intended) is not "pro-life": it is certainly not pro-love.

I speak of this, not only as a theologian and an ethicist but as a pastor. How often I have attended to people who wished to have children but could not and, in a few instances, women who worked through very difficult pregnancies, sometimes spending months in bed in order to make a healthy delivery possible. In two or three instances, either the pregnancy was not sustainable or the baby was unable to survive. In two such cases, the next pregnancy was altogether different. Sometimes I wish the so-called "pro life" advocates could see the deeply spiritual dimensions of this and know that real love of life means taking the realities seriously into account. Incidentally, I speak of this not only as a theologian, an ethicist and a pastor, but also as a grandfather. And you need to know that this Sunday I am to baptize our latest granddaughter, born into a home where she is deeply cherished and where she will receive the nurturing for her to grow into womanhood as the person God intends her to be.

Simple justice

Whatever the mode of making family, one thing is clear. The psychological relief of having choices has changed the landscape of family formation and the dynamics of sexual power in America. Now, women, too, can enjoy their sexuality without fear of pregnancy, as men always have been able to do. Being able to make love without making babies is a prerequisite to a satisfying sexual relationship but even more to a marriage of true equals. Similarly, when infertility occurs, a woman valued by society and her family for her own self is not cast aside as she would have been in earlier times and still can be in some corners of the world. When men and women are equal partners in all life's endeavors, we are truly moving toward a world of responsible choices and planned, wanted children.

For only when equals come together can both men and women be free to follow their hearts and their minds in making the families that are right for them. The freedom of equal power, of functional rather than rigid roles, of open and honest communication about sexuality, is the freedom to make family in the twenty-first century in fulfilling ways not dreamed of in earlier eras.

I am blessed with such a marriage, with such a life partner. Though we have given birth to no children together, we have blended our families into a new mix that is enriched by each member and woven into a whole cloth by love. Together, we share our own family values that I believe represent the best of humanity: respect for those who think, act, believe differently from us; equality of race, sex, age, sexual orientation; and freedom to consider and the power to act upon all life's choices.

Others have different ways of making family and that's the point. Thanks to the reproductive rights movement, these quiet, individual choices can be made out of love, not fear, and out of hope, not despair.

Family planning was perhaps the greatest advance for social justice in the twentieth century because it affects everyone, male or female, young and old. My way of making family and your way of making family stand as living, loving proof.

Chapter 8

Choice as sacrifice, choice as freedom
Or, how I became a perfect ten

❋ I did the thing I felt was best for all of us and sent them back to heaven.

❋ Successful, still together and eagerly awaiting a baby that we *planned*.

❋ I found there are many ways to be a mother in this world without having biological children.

Three people, three choices, three slices of life in all its richness and diversity.

A new look at the meaning of reproductive choice

People often assume that a personal experience with abortion motivated me to become a passionate advocate for reproductive choice. But it is a lot more complicated than that, as are most women's stories about their lives. For every choice has its parallel choices known but not taken. When I was fifteen and pregnant, I was aware that the option of abortion existed even though it was illegal. I chose not to go that route. Like so many women, I did not choose adoption. This doesn't mean these are not entirely valid choices. I just knew they weren't right for me. I wanted children and thought I was ready for parenthood. I even thought I wanted four children until I had three and was physically exhausted.

When I was thirty-two, after twelve years of taking the high-dose birth control pills that were available then, my body was starting to rebel. The only solution I could see was sterilization. I was not really ready to foreclose my fertility; still, it seemed the best option at the time. By and by, I became divorced from my first husband. By and by, I met the love of my life, Alex Barbanell, and we married in 1980. We each had three wonderful children already. From the standpoint of responsibility toward world population, we had certainly done our part. I was never highly motivated enough to try to reverse the tubal ligation. If, however, there is one great sadness for me, it is that I have never had the pleasure of having a truly planned child with someone I wholeheartedly love and at a time of life when we could have provided the environment in which a child could have the best chance to thrive.

Don't people understand that when faced with an unintended pregnancy, or a situation like I found myself in at thirty-two when I chose sterilization, all the choices available are imperfect and fraught with pain?

Choice is freedom, yes, but choice is also sacrifice. For in the very act of choosing, we are relinquishing our claim to the other options. This is never truer than when the issue is childbearing, when the path we choose defines our very lives. When the choice of one path may preclude forever the taking of the others. When the choice has such a profound impact on those we love the most.

Many choices, many reasons

 At eighteen, I chose to bring my daughter into this world, one of the toughest choices I had to make. I look at her and am thankful every day. Then about six months ago, it was confirmed that I was pregnant again. Looking at my life, the struggles I've had to endure to make sure my daughter was fed well and taken care of, I knew that another child was not a feasible thing at this time in my life. I had an abortion. I look back and I know that I made the right choice. It was a hard choice, just as deciding to keep my little girl was. Now I still have a chance of making my daughter's life a successful one.

—Nell, age twenty-two

 At sixteen weeks, routine prenatal screening tests came back incredibly abnormal. Two weeks, many tests, and sleepless nights filled with dread later we got the news that our baby was fatally ill with an extremely rare genetic disease. At eighteen weeks, we terminated our much-wanted pregnancy at the hospital where we planned to give birth. Our risk of losing another baby to this terrible disease is one in four. But two years later, I'm happy to tell you I'm the proud mom of a beautiful, healthy baby boy. Choice is still there for me, ensuring that if I ever have another affected pregnancy that I will also have choices.

—Lucie, age thirty-three

 I was twenty-four years old when I became pregnant. I was ill with Panic Disorder & OCD [Obsessive-Complusive Disorder]. I was always afraid I was losing my mind. My husband was a substance abuser, abusive to me, and we lived in poverty. After much soul searching, I decided on an abortion. I hadn't any idea how to keep a child safe; I couldn't even keep myself safe. After the abortion, I had the fortitude and courage to leave my husband. There are many reasons that women need the right to choose, among them: physical and mental illness, poverty, abuse, sex that was forced upon them, sex that they were coerced into. I have found there are many ways to be a mother in this world, without having biological children.

—Cecile, age forty

This happily married mother of two in the following story, with her husband already scheduled for a vasectomy, discovered that she was pregnant, and she and her husband decided to have an abortion—at first.

 It was not a decision my husband or I took lightly, and we weighed our options at great length before making this painful choice. While waiting the week for our appointment, we ended up changing our minds. We decided that adding to our family could have some advantages, and that we could try to rearrange our lives in order to have another child. Even though we decided to continue this pregnancy, I thank God and all people who have fought for my right to decide what is right for me and my family.

—Jane, age thirty-nine

Looking through the moral prism

Making decisions about pregnancy and childbearing is like looking into a prism from different angles and seeing the issues differently each time, depending on your vantage point.

 When I told my parents I was pregnant they tried to force me to have an abortion, but I decided to proceed with the pregnancy. Today, I am so glad that I decided to have my son, but I strongly believe that my case is an exception to the rule. I was in a very stable relationship with a man I knew I would someday marry, I came from a wealthy family who offers much needed emotional and financial support, and I am almost through with college.

—Tina, age twenty

I was an avid believer that abortions were 100 percent wrong and I would never do such a thing. Being adopted I could not help but think that my biological mother could have done the same thing to me. After going to the doctor and discussing the situation with my boyfriend I decided I did not want this child. [Her regular doctor told her that he couldn't accommodate her for an abortion. He offered her prenatal care instead.] My experience gave me a chance to feel what it is like to have no say in the matter of what you want to do with your child. Fortunately, I was able to go to a clinic for an abortion.

—Abby, age nineteen

 My mother had an abortion when her and my father were first married. They were not ready for a child. She was very ill at the time, and childbirth would not have made that any easier. If she hadn't made the choice to have that abortion, I may never have been born.

—Onice, age twenty-five

 I don't believe in abortion unless it's a rape or molestation case. I believe that there shouldn't be a choice; the person makes that choice when they have sex. I guess I might have different feelings if I was in that situation.

—Geoff, age thirty

Where you stand, as they say, depends on where you sit. And the way real life works, where you sit today will inevitably change tomorrow. So it stands to reason that the principled choices we make will be influenced as we take into account the factors and values of particular situations. One commonsensical, but often overlooked, fact is that different choices are right at different times of life. I am struck by how some of the most powerful stories come from people who have experienced multiple choices and talk about how the "right" choice changes with the life cycle, like these four stories:

Different choices for different times

 Nine years ago my long term boyfriend and I discovered I was pregnant. After many sleepless nights and emotional discussions, we decided that the best *choice* for our future was to terminate the pregnancy. In the years since, I have frequently thought of our choice and while I wish it hadn't had to be made in the first place, I *know* we did the right thing for us. Today, we are still together, have been married for two years and are expecting our first baby in March. I feel very strongly that had we not had the right to make that choice, we would not be where we are today. Successful, still together and eagerly awaiting a baby that we *planned*. This is an issue that I feel strongly about.

—Maggie, age twenty-nine

 I was very embarrassed by this unplanned, unwanted pregnancy that was a result of carelessness. I decided to tell no one of my decision and to go alone. Most of my family is pro-life. I have always been pro-choice. I do feel abortion is wrong, but I also know that a lot of things are wrong in this world—especially the fact that men are just not always physically, emotionally and/or financially responsible for the children they help produce. In my case I am a mature woman (thirty-seven) and a single mother to a toddler. Although my son would benefit from a sibling I felt we would both benefit the most from my own sanity. I wasn't prepared to go through this pregnancy alone, and to live exhausted and possibly very poor for the first few years of this child's life. I'm already a single mother—I'm already tired—and I already have a child in this world who needs all of my time and attention. After much prayer and thought, I just felt I couldn't take on more responsibility without a devoted partner!!!

—Jeanne, age thirty-seven

 Reproductive choice made the difference for our family. My husband (of now 14 years) and I had only begun our relationship almost twenty years ago when we had a contraceptive failure (gotta love your diaphragm!). We were both medical students, just at the beginning of our careers. Neither of us was ready in any way to start a family and both of us had great ambitions for our careers. After great thought, we aborted. We stayed together and worked hard on our relationship, and med school. We completed our residency in family medicine, then spent a year in Asia, where we volunteered at a clinic in Nepal. We returned to the states, a very solid couple and ten years after our first pregnancy we chose to start a family. We now have two beautiful, delightful, very loved children (ages four and eight), and we work part-time (so that we can both spend time with our children) in a community clinic providing care for the indigent population. Our family is thriving, and our relationship is solid because we had the time and opportunity to create a stable foundation before starting our family. Now that I have kids, and know the stress involved in raising children I am so grateful to have had the opportunity to create my family when we were ready.

—Sharon, early forties

 The first time I became pregnant was at the age of seventeen and a half. I got pregnant the first time I ever had sex. The encounter was with a married military man, considerably older than I. At that time, I was not on any method of birth control. The pregnancy was truly unintended, the whole act of intercourse was not intended. Now that this had happened, a choice had to be made. I chose to have my child and place him up for adoption immediately after his birth. This was undoubtedly the single hardest decision, and experience, of my life thus far. I will live forever with the knowledge that there is a human being out there, part of my flesh and blood, that I may never know and never see. I find this difficult to live with day to day. It has been almost thirteen years, and I remember every day of my pregnancy, his delivery, the adoption process as if it were yesterday. But I had a choice, and made that choice. Several years later, I was involved in a relationship with an abusive man. He was abusive mentally, physically and sexually. I felt there was no way I was going through the adoption route again, and I couldn't see myself having a child with this man. Abortion was my choice. It was hard decision, but one that I could make comfortably and live with myself. I feel that I have seen all sides of the controversy and have enacted two of these three possible solution scenarios. I am comfortable with all of the decisions I have made and thank the higher power that we, as women, have the ability, the capability and the resources to choose what works best for *us*. The government doesn't tell a man what to do with his penis.

—Winnie, age thirty

Trust women to understand life's choices

Politicians and anti-choice demagogues often tout adoption as the solution to all unintended pregnancies, forgetting (if they ever knew) that each person's circumstance is unique and that each woman's life has value and purpose independent of her reproductive life.

Every girl or woman who becomes pregnant understands that there are childless couples interested in adoption and agencies that will help her through the pregnancy and the process. But only a very small number of women, 2-to-3 percent who have unintended pregnancies, choose that option. Some who choose adoption are completely at peace with their decision. Some write to me expressing the deep sadness that haunts them every day. Many write to explain why adoption wasn't for them. As with all reproductive choices, these varied decisions are complex, heartfelt, and deeply moral.

 My story is very simple. I got pregnant at the age of sixteen. I never expected that it would happen to me. I knew that I would not be able to have the babies and be strong enough to give them away. I also knew that there was no way that I would raise my children as a burden to me and society. Therefore, I did the thing that I felt was best for all of us and sent them back to heaven. Now that I am older I wish that I would have been able to give them the life that they deserve. But since that would not have been possible, I am so thankful for having the option. I probably would have found a way to get an abortion, but since they are legal, then I was given the opportunity to have a safe and effective one.

—Alia, age twenty-four

No food, no money, and no one to care for me. I was raped and ended up pregnant. I went through with the pregnancy and had a beautiful little girl. I named her Elisabeth, and planned on keeping her, but there was one problem . . . I still had no home and it was almost winter. I gave her up for adoption. It was a closed adoption . . . now I can't see my daughter until she turns eighteen, that is fifteen years from now! I can only see her then if she comes and finds me, I am not allowed to look for her. It is hard to get through every day, but I am still glad I gave her up, so she wouldn't have to live the life I had to.

—Shannon, age sixteen

Passions run high about reproductive choices because they are so profoundly personal. Businessman John Martinson wrote the following letter describing how a friend became stridently anti-choice after becoming a parent through adoption. John, himself an adoptive parent, takes a more generous view:

 During the interview with the birth mother, I told her I support women's rights and reproductive freedom, and I would raise a boy to respect women and to treat them as equals. I believe this was a key part of her decision to select us. We were excited to share the news, especially with my close friend who had adopted two kids some years before. After the adoption of his first child, my friend changed. He became very angry and resentful of my support of choice. It became something we could not discuss. I hoped that would change when he received my e-mail with our good news.

His response was mean-spirited and resentful. "You will be in our prayers. You should thank God she didn't choose abortion." After I recovered from the hurt, I shot back the following response: "I know we will never agree on this, but you should know why I am passionate about a woman's right to choose. This is an intensely personal decision by a woman in consultation with her doctor. And it is *her* decision . . . not the state's. Women can never be free as long as the state attempts to control her pregnancy. I don't thank God she didn't choose abortion, I thank her. If she had chosen abortion, there are many others around the world who choose adoption for their babies every day. And there are not enough adoptive parents to adopt them all. You and I have known each other a very long time. I respect your right to believe the way you do. Please respect my right to believe as I do. Let us just agree to disagree as we have in the past."

I never got a response. Now we have a five-and-one-half-month-old bouncing baby boy and I have never been more supportive of a woman's right to choose.

People often express moral ambivalence in their childbearing choices, whether abortion, adoption, or parenting. We must respect their ability both to make these choices and to comprehend, value, and even mourn for what they did not choose.

Robbie Ausley, an Austin, Texas, mother of four whom you met earlier, tells her story:

 Having healthy twin daughters on my twenty-seventh birthday in 1971 was certainly a surprise and a blessing. I did, however, find myself in the hospital worrying about being a good mother to all four of my young children. I had grown up in a large, loving family with three older brothers and had fond memories of those childhood days. However, because my husband worked long hours, I became the primary caretaker and emotional parent of our children. Sometimes I felt like a plucked hen, desperately wishing there was more of me to go around.

Then in 1973 when the twins were two, we were faced with what I perceived to be a catastrophic dilemma. Tom's vasectomy of two years failed, and I was pregnant again! I immediately called Tom and insisted that I was incapable of nurturing and sustaining another baby. He attempted to calm my fears by suggesting we add an extra room onto the house and hire a live-in nanny. "But you don't understand," I reacted, "money cannot change the fact that I am their mother, and there is only one of me to fulfill that significant role." We spent the next week praying about our dilemma and seeking counsel with professionals, including our minister. Ultimately Tom and I made what we believed to be a life-affirming, moral decision within the context of our faith—and that was to terminate the pregnancy.

Two strongly held convictions have stayed with me since that experience over twenty-eight years ago. First, it made me fully aware of the realization that we don't live in a perfect world. If we did, Tom and I would not have been faced with such a difficult decision. However, I feel strongly that I was in the best position and therefore the best person to ultimately make that decision. Not even Tom, the person who knew me best and loved me most, could understand the depth of my anxiety nor the gravity of my emotional, mental health.

The second impression I still have etched in my heart and soul is the desperateness and level of panic I felt that day when the doctor called. I remember locking myself in my bedroom, the three younger ones crying and banging on the door as I hysterically cried on the phone, pleading with Tom to take me somewhere to get an abortion—I did not care where but I had to do something because I had these four precious, innocent children depending on me. Therefore, my second strongly held conviction is that women, regardless of their financial status, will find a way to get an abortion, even if it means endangering their lives.

I continued to be a "stay-at-home" mom, fully committed to nurturing all four children into adulthood with the hope that they would one day contribute to the society in which we live. Today, all four children seem to be well-adjusted adults: college-educated, married, and with children of their own. Because of my personal journey, the bumper sticker on my car reads, "Pro-faith, pro-family, pro-choice."

Almost everybody is, to some degree, pro-choice

To help people clarify their views about abortion, I often do an exercise that asks them to place themselves along a hypothetical continuum ranging from one to ten—one being all abortions are murder and should be outlawed; ten being the decision about abortion should always be up to the woman.

We find virtually no one ever claims to be a "one." Very few people would choose to save the life of the fetus over the life of the woman.

Most people position themselves somewhere between four and eight. Every individual who does this exercise can explain the circumstances (life of woman, rape, health, mental health, social well-being, etc.) that make abortion acceptable in his or her moral framework. So almost everyone is pro-choice. Only the degree varies. Once the discussion starts, people often move from place to place on the continuum as they think more deeply about the issues involved. Their movement is usually toward the higher numbers as people reflect on the complexity of the issues.

As a result of my personal experiences, I am a perfect ten—against any laws that restrict access to the full range of a woman's reproductive choices.

I believe all of life's choices are difficult. None is perfect in its consequences, so one has no right to judge another's reproductive choices. You can attribute my conviction to rational thought and research. But I am more inclined to credit it to simple experience with some of those choices. It makes you humble. That's why, regardless of my choices, I would over the long-term place my faith in women to make the best decisions for themselves and their offspring. Because I know from my own experience and the stories of so many thousands of women and men that choice is indeed freedom. But it is also always sacrifice.

Part III
Personally political

I am so grateful and thankful for the rights and choices I have been given because of the battles fought by other women. While some of my teenaged friends were affected by unwanted pregnancies in the 1980s, I was fortunate enough to have protection and kept my pride. They had wonderful counseling and were offered choices to decide what was best for them personally and morally. They had access to abortion.

Males can have immediate abortion on demand just by turning their backs and walking away. Stricter child support doesn't solve the problem because the men who want to be involved in the child's life are the ones who are there and already pay. The simple fact is that a man will never be affected by this issue the way women are. I marched in Washington D.C. with thousands of others to protect our right to free choice while I was in college. I hope to have a baby in the near future now that I am ready and I am so thankful for the bright, strong, courageous women who came before me. I also can't stress enough how important it is to *vote!* I always do. Make sure your candidate supports families and *choice!*

—Ashley, age thirty-six

Chapter Nine

Viagra® yes, birth control no

My first awareness of racial injustice came at age three, when I became morally outraged that Juanita, my favorite babysitter, couldn't go to the high school on "our" side of town. I was a child of the South, and racial discrimination suffused the culture so completely that most people couldn't even see it. I'll admit that my outrage was fueled by the knowledge that when school started, she would have to go live with her grandmother across town and therefore wouldn't be available to play with me. Even so, this incident stayed with me. I am sure that Juanita's plight shaped my sensibilities about fairness and justice, or the lack of it, in this world.

Like racial injustice in the South fifty years ago, other injustices are so pervasive that many don't see them until somebody points them out. That's exactly what happened with the pervasive gender inequities in women's health care, not the least of which is the absence of insurance coverage for contraception under many plans. But unlike the complex issues of race, religion, and culture, once this injustice was pointed out, people "got" it very quickly.

I was absolutely appalled at the media attention given to Viagra, and then to hear about it being covered by medical insurance; the same kind that wouldn't pay for my yearly female physical, or my choice to use a single prescription that would allow me to prevent pregnancy. Sometimes I still can't believe in the injustice of health issues women still have today, and how degrading it is to us. One can only wonder: how will insurers handle the new male birth control that will be available in five years? I guarantee there will not be this level of debate or controversy, mark my words.

—Michelle, age thirty-two

 I have health insurance but it does not cover women's health at all.
—anonymous patient

I am a wife and mother. I also teach fourth grade. I had almost reached a state of depression when I found out that my insurance would not cover my birth control pills, unless needed for medical reasons. I am a newlywed and a new mother. During this time I cannot risk having another child nor deny my husband or myself marital pleasure. I was paying an extra $30 per month on birth control pills. It was just too much to handle with the new four hundred dollars per month child care, baby formula, and clothing.

—B. J., thirties

Jennifer Erickson confronts an injustice

Jennifer Erickson was a newlywed Seattle pharmacist working for Bartell Drug Company. She had no notion of herself as an activist for a cause. But Jennifer came face-to-face with the gender injustice of insurance plans that cover most other drugs but not contraception—and the personal became political as a result of her first-hand experience, both as a woman and a health care professional.

I consider myself in many ways a typical American woman. My husband Scott and I have been married for two years. We recently bought our first house. Someday when we feel ready, Scott and I would like to have one or two children. Like many Americans, I get my health insurance through my employer. Shortly after I started working there, I discovered that the company health plan did not cover contraception. Personally, it was very disappointing for me, since contraception is my most important, ongoing health need at this time.

But it was also troubling to me professionally, as a health care provider. Contraception is one of the most common prescriptions I fill for women. I am often the person who has the difficult job of telling a woman that her insurance plan will not cover contraceptives. I am unable to give her an acceptable explanation. Why? Because there is no acceptable explanation for this shortsighted policy. My perspective from behind the pharmacy counter gives me a clear picture of the burden this policy places on women, especially the low-income women who are the least equipped to deal with an unplanned pregnancy. I have seen women leave the pharmacy empty-handed because they cannot afford to pay the full cost of their birth control pills, and it breaks my heart.

In 1996, we found only one-third of indemnity insurance plans covered the birth control pill. Fewer yet covered all medically approved methods of birth control. And because women are so determined to get those pills—to control their fertility—they pay up. That $30 a month (for oral contraceptives) is a significant part of the reason that women pay 68 percent more than men out-of-pocket for health care. More recently, in 2001, the Kaiser Family Foundation found that only one-third of self-insured employer plans cover the pill.

Jennifer, for one, was fed up with the view from her pharmacy counter. She says:

I finally got tired of telling women "no this is one prescription your insurance won't cover." So I took the bold step of bringing a lawsuit against my employer to challenge its unfair policy.

The sexes are unequal when it comes to their reproductive equipment. Women have most of it, and they have the part that not only needs frequent medical maintenance but can ruin their health or even kill them without appropriate care. Basically, it's well-woman health care, which includes things like Pap smears to check for cancer or precancerous cells. This care, plus the contraceptive methods that enable women to plan and space their childbearing, constitutes most of the health care women need during their fertile years. Many insurance plans ignore this care, and even those that cover the exams often fail to cover the contraceptives.

This reminds me of the old story of the pig and the chicken, who were walking past a restaurant advertising bacon and eggs for breakfast. "Sounds all right," said the chicken. "Maybe all right for you," replied the pig. "For you, it's just a contribution. But for me, it's a total commitment."

For women, pregnancy *is* a total commitment. And yet insurance plans often treat the medical means to decide whether and when to have a pregnancy as though they were frivolous luxuries—instead of significant necessities. Women like those cited below have described their situations on www.covermypills.com.

 Our health plan, like most others does not cover the pill. When I confronted our provider they had no explanation. However, they did say that they would cover a vasectomy or a hysterectomy. We had just had our second child and we had not yet decided if we would have a third. To have such a drastic procedure done that I might regret later was not a concern to the insurance company. I feel that the type of birth control a person uses is a personal choice. I feel that it is unfair for the insurance companies to make that decision for us. Worse yet, to push us into a decision whether or not to have another child. These decisions take time and thought.

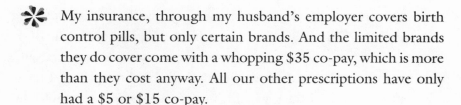 My insurance, through my husband's employer covers birth control pills, but only certain brands. And the limited brands they do cover come with a whopping $35 co-pay, which is more than they cost anyway. All our other prescriptions have only had a $5 or $15 co-pay.

I have been on birth control for two years and my husband's insurance does not cover my pills so for two years I have been paying about thirty dollars a month on a prescription that is needed. I have two children and my last child has a lot of medical illness and I would like to prevent getting pregnant right now until we know for sure if this is genetic or not so our family has been struggling not only to pay for medical attention but to prevent pregnancies.

How we're fixing the problem

There is progress on this front because the injustices are now being pointed out and people are paying attention. Early in 1997, I met with Senator Olympia Snowe (R-ME) and she immediately agreed to be a primary sponsor for what would be the Equity in Prescription Insurance and Contraceptive Coverage Act (EPICC). We drafted legislation and built a broad coalition in Congress—led by Snowe, a pro-choice Republican and Senator Harry Reid, an anti-choice Democrat from Nevada—that could support the basic fairness of insurance coverage for the medical care that prevents unintended pregnancy. After all, it just makes sense that if you oppose abortion, you ought to support access to contraception that prevents abortion from ever being an issue.

Sometimes controversy can work in your favor, and this was certainly one of those times. Bob Dole and Viagra helped by making the issue, well, sexy. Similar legislation already was moving in California when we started this effort. But federal legislation for contraceptive equity languished in Congress for several years—until the word got out that plans quickly began covering Viagra while still not covering contraception. This triggered outrage from the grassroots. The obvious injustice that men's sexual performance was considered more valuable than women's reproductive health really riled people up. I knew we were on the right track when no insurance companies would debate publicly against the legislation. Pretty soon you could feel the nationwide groundswell. We took on the debate and focused it on the impact these long-standing inequities have on the lives of individual women like Jennifer, the young pharmacist.

More and more states—twenty and counting—are requiring insurance companies within their borders to cover contraceptives if they cover other prescription drugs. Federal employees now are guaranteed coverage—and President George W. Bush got his hand slapped when he tried to change that by taking it out of his budget. But in spite of the outcry, federal legislation—the Equity in Prescription Insurance and Contraceptive Coverage Act—that applies to insurance plans across the board still hasn't passed. So we added to the effort another strategy—lawsuits, such as Jennifer's courageous litigation, that can help improve the lives of individuals and signal to companies and legislators that the courts reject this inequity.

Birth control is basic health care and access to it is gender equity, plain and simple

In June 2001, Jennifer won her class-action lawsuit, assuring coverage for all the women who work for her company and putting employers everywhere on notice. Similar lawsuits are now springing up in other locations.

More and more women are speaking out

❋ I worked as a pharmacy technician for two years. Other than women that were receiving low-cost contraceptives via state aid, very few women had the co-pay or option of having discounted contraceptive prescriptions. I found it extremely difficult to explain to women why their prescription wasn't covered and why men's Viagra was. These women, whether they were trying to avoid pregnancy, dealing with ovarian cysts, endometriosis, etc. were never allowed the right to receive the care that they deserved. It's infuriating to dispense Viagra to a middle-aged man with a $5 co-pay when his only condition is the fact that he can't get an erection! A woman's quality of life is more affected by disease or childbirth than a man that has difficulty becoming aroused!

—Anne, age thirty

❋ I am an employer (female) with a small business of six women. First we had to battle to find a decent healthcare plan (which costs a fortune, but is worth it). Then we had to battle for coverage of contraception. We were told that our plan would cover contraception if deemed "medically necessary." Our first medically necessary claim has been denied. The moral: there are employers who want to add contraception, but can't because of the plans available to small business owners.

—Nan, age fifty-five

❋ About six months ago I switched HMO's. I was astonished to learn from my pharmacist that coverage for my birth control prescription had been denied. When I called the company the customer service representative told me that New York state was not required to cover my prescription and would only do so if it was a "medical necessity". I then asked if my policy would cover an abortion. I was told "*Yes*"! Furiously I growled back "You mean you won't pay for me to avoid getting pregnant, but you'll pay for me to not be pregnant?" Again I was told "*Yes*"! After hanging up I felt a huge amount of anger and personal violation. I had never felt so discriminated against solely because of my gender. I quickly fired off e-mails to my senators and other representatives and sent a letter to my insurance company.

—Kathleen, age thirty-two

But it's not over yet. Here's what Jennifer Erickson told a recent U.S. Senate hearing on contraceptive insurance coverage:

 Despite our victory in federal court, I know that my case is not enough to help all of the American women who need this essential health care. At this point, my case is directly binding only on Bartell. Nearly every day one of my customers thanks me for coming forward and congratulates me on winning the case; but many of the women I serve at my pharmacy counter *still* do not have insurance coverage for the contraception *they* need. But I also know that Title VII, the anti discrimination law that my case is based on, doesn't cover all women. And, even more important, women should not have to file federal court lawsuits to get their basic health care needs covered.

So today I am speaking for millions of American women who want to time their pregnancies and welcome their children into the world when they are ready. On behalf of the women of this Nation, I urge you to enact this comprehensive legislation, because every woman, no matter what state she lives in or where she works, should have fair access to the method of contraception she needs.

I will not soon forget the exhilaration I felt after that long, hot day in Seneca Falls, New York, where we were celebrating the 150th anniversary of the women's movement. I arrived home from the events just in time to get a call from an excited colleague telling me to turn on *C-Span* right away. I found the U. S. House of Representatives debating the question of contraceptive coverage for federal employees. After one-hundred-and-fifty years. My tears flowed at the significance of this historic moment. Congresswoman Nita Lowey (D-NY) was speaking brilliantly in support of the measure. Behind her was a multicolored sea of skirts—women of both political parties united in support of this basic women's health care measure. When Representative Chris Smith (R-NJ) rose to oppose the legislation because he regards some methods of birth control as abortifacients, Representative Nancy Johnson (R-CT) gave an impassioned rebuttal:

 Is there no limit to my colleague's willingness to impose his concept of when life begins on others? . . . [This] reflects a level of intrusion into conscience, into independence, into freedom, that, frankly, I have never witnessed.

A model for pro-choice policy initiatives

Stay tuned. We are going to remedy this injustice in every state, in every company, for every woman in every insurance plan. And we're going to tackle other similar issues—such as the refusal clauses that allow pharmacists to refuse to fill prescriptions for birth control methods, even when they are the only provider in town. We will take on any injustice where the right to determine when and whether to have children is rendered hollow by societal, financial, and other barriers.

All of this activism didn't just happen. In fact, it has taken years of gathering information, educating, and organizing. But the progress that has been made toward rectifying the gender injustice of the lack of contraceptive coverage can be a model for future progress toward universal access to all reproductive health care. Possibly even more important than the results of the work that has been done to ensure contraceptive coverage—as vital as that is—is the sea change this campaign represents in how the reproductive rights movement thinks about its agenda.

It's the difference between a thermometer and a thermostat. A thermometer is a gauge of the climate. A thermostat controls the climate. By advancing policies that bring about universal access to reproductive health care, we can control the climate of reproductive rights and health care in this country. It takes a four-pronged strategy—of legislation, communication, litigation, and mobilization—to be the nation's reproductive rights thermostat. But in doing so, we operate from a climate of great strength because the stories of real women's lives bear compelling witness to the fact that these policies are right and just.

Here's a good example: until about twenty years ago, medical research usually involved male-only studies, but assumed or implied that the results could also be applied to women, too. Thanks to concerted lobbying efforts by women's groups such as the National Black Women's Health project and the National Women's Health Network, women are now included in research on a more equitable basis. And gender-specific research such as breast cancer and hormone replacement therapy now receive their fair share of government research funds.

Maybe someday I won't get any more letters like these:

 In 1992 I was diagnosed by my gynecologist with a "menstrual dysfunction." This was due to having a 96 day cycle. Yes a 96 day cycle. At the time I was working for a bank and as long as I had a note from my doctor HMO would cover the prescription. All I had to pay was my co-pay amount. However two years ago I switched jobs and my new employer does not cover the "Pill." Even though it was prescribed for medical purposes. I am currently paying $29.95 a month to keep myself regulated. I cannot understand why my current insurance company will not cover me. However, a girl that I work with was put on the "pill" for medical purposes and she is covered under her husband's medical plan. Also, one of the girls in the office is now pregnant. The insurance will cover all of her "pregnancy," but will not cover the two of us with medical problems.

—Janet, age thirty-eight

 It's not so much the fact that the insurance company doesn't claim to offer contraceptives—they do. The problem is that they conveniently placed birth control pills in the highest co-pay bracket of $35, when pills cost about $31 at the pharmacy. What the company I work for is doing is setting up what is called a Section 125 so that employees can have money held from their checks before taxes and put in a fund to cover medications the insurance company doesn't cover. This will help but it still does not excuse the insurance company for increasing the co-pay to an amount that is higher than the price of the pills.

—Beth, age twenty-nine

I asked Jennifer Erickson why she was so generously willing to give her available time off from her job and the great amount of energy it had taken her to be the plaintiff in a major lawsuit. She told me that she really hadn't set out to be any kind of a symbol. She had merely become tired of customers yelling at her as a pharmacist because their insurance didn't cover contraceptives. And personally she thought it was only fair that her company's insurance should cover contraceptives—they are, after all, in the health care business.

"But what I didn't anticipate," she said, "is that it feels really good to help so many people. Sometimes it just blows me away"—at this point her tears begin to flow—"that it will help so many people for so many years to come."

Chapter Ten

Rights v. access

A three-hour drive

 My mother, who had an abortion in 1976, assumed that abortion would remain safe and legal forever. She experienced a rude awakening when I came home from college for summer break in 1998 asking for her help as I faced an unplanned pregnancy. As she searched for an abortion provider, she realized the damage that abortion rights had suffered since her youth. While we traveled three hours to another state to access a provider, she apologized for her generation's complacency concerning reproductive rights.

I may have a daughter someday, and I never want to have that conversation with her. Not that I would be devastated if she found herself pregnant and considering abortion, just like her mother and grandmother had many years ago. I simply could not watch her struggle to find a provider in another state. I will not watch the complacency of my generation allow abortion rights to disappear completely.

—Susan, age twenty-three

I hope this writer's commitment continues, because the reproductive rights and health movement needs her passion and her advocacy. She understands what so many others who think we can't go back to the bad old days don't yet get: the bad old days are here.

Rights without access are meaningless

All right, *Roe v. Wade* hasn't been overturned; abortion isn't illegal. *Griswold v. Connecticut,* which legalized birth control and established the precedent of a right to privacy in reproductive decisions, stands. But our state and federal lawmakers, our courts, and our society's lack of respect for women and children have ensured that many of us do not have the information, resources, or access to make those rights real. And rights without access are meaningless. If present trends continue, *"Access Denied"* may as well be stamped on the door of reproductive health centers.

If you're poor, or young, or are in the military, or live in rural America, you technically have the right to a legal abortion. But you'll have to climb over barriers of distance, judicial review, transportation, money, waiting periods, mandated biased propaganda that encourages childbirth over abortion, and more to try to get one. The result might be a more expensive, more difficult, delayed abortion or one like Becky Bell's, the Indiana teen whose death is a chilling reminder of life before *Roe v. Wade.*

For military women, or dependents, it could mean an abortion in a foreign hospital in a foreign country because the medical facilities on U.S. bases can't do abortions, even if you pay for it yourself. And what if you're stationed in a country where, unlike the country you are putting your life on the line to serve, abortion is illegal?

If your employer pays your medical bills, you may have to pay out of pocket for contraceptives like Jennifer Erickson used to have to do, before her successful lawsuit; like Elizabeth Dole might have to were she of childbearing age, while Bob gets his Viagra for free. If your pharmacist sees fit to judge your choices, your prescription for emergency contraception might not be filled. If the only hospital in your rural town just merged into a Catholic system, your tubal ligation, or other emergency medical needs may be a three-hour drive away.

 A lot of doctors will not prescribe ECP [emergency contraception pills], and they may not understand your situation and they don't really want to.

—Randi, age twenty-three

At the age of seventeen, I was raped by my neighbor. My immediate feelings were of such numbness, and fear that I wasn't thinking straight and I couldn't even think of what to do. My friend encouraged me to go to Student Health for the morning-after pill and I did first thing Monday morning. Even though the doctor looked at me like an irresponsible college girl sleeping around and needing emergency contraception because I couldn't yet speak about what had happened to me, having access to the pill saved my life. I don't know what I would have done if I had become pregnant with my rapist's baby. I was in such shock and fear that I don't know what I would have done to myself if I had become pregnant.

—Sunitra, age twenty-two

Access to abortion is often nonexistent for women who rely on Medicaid for their health insurance, and this has been so since Representative Henry Hyde began attacking these services soon after abortion became legal. As a result, the federal government now sits in judgment of low-income women facing unintended pregnancies. This has created a gap in women's health care where abortion services should, by rights and good medical practice, be routinely included.

Charity alone is not sufficient to close this gap, though many kind and generous donors routinely open their checkbooks as well as their hearts to women who plead for assistance. No one in America should have to plead for health care, most especially health care so basic as reproductive health care. Inconvenience, expense, delays—in what other area of health care is access so severely restricted? It is another injustice that, when pointed out, brings the kind of outrage that fuels revolution.

Doctors fight back

The story of the founding of Medical Students for Choice is a heartening example of just such a revolution, one from inside the healing profession itself which is helping to restore access to abortion services. And it is an example of what a small group of citizens can accomplish when they decide to take action. The background: sure, abortion is legal. But what does that mean when the majority of doctors who perform abortions are over the age of sixty-five? We've already heard it means a three-hour drive. After years of harassment and violence against doctors, U.S. medical schools in the 1990s acted as if the most common outpatient procedure for women barely existed. The majority of obstetrics and gynecology residency programs didn't require basic instruction on how to perform abortions or counsel women with unintended pregnancies.

But the anti-choice folks overplayed their hand when they sent gruesome pictures to medical student Jody Steinauer. She was outraged, and immediately called the National Abortion Federation to see what she could do. She went to work for them and founded Medical Students for Choice, a group that has lobbied successfully to return abortion to medical school curricula. In a very short time, they estimate they have made changes in at least one-third of the medical schools in the U.S. Just a few committed individuals, combined with a just cause and the ability to spread the word to the grassroots, have made a big difference.

Information is power. When I was in high school, I knew where the bootlegger lived in our "dry" town. The boys went there to buy beer regularly and it was no big secret. But birth control? I knew from the book my father had given me that it existed. The boys carried condoms in their pockets and the glove compartments of their cars, but I had no idea where they got them. I vaguely remember knowing about diaphragms. I have no idea if or what kind of birth control my mother used, but she obviously spaced her children. My grandmother used to say she wished she had had four children instead of two, and I now wonder how she managed to have just two.

When your choices conflict with your hospital's religion

But information alone isn't enough. In our health care system, the gatekeepers can deny access financially and practically when your choices and beliefs conflict with theirs. As these writers can attest:

 I have a female relative who works for a social service agency which is operated by the Catholic Archdiocese. Last month, all employees received a memo informing them about upcoming changes in their health insurance benefits. One of the changes is that all family planning (birth control, etc.) will be excluded from their benefit package. The Foundation openly admits that this is being done solely because of the Catholic Church's opposition to any and all forms of birth control. I wonder how far this would go if this was a Jewish organization, and all the male employees were required to be circumcised?

—Jeanie, age thirty-seven

 I had asked prior to taking the job about the religious beliefs of the diocese, which partially funded some of the programs at the agency. I was told that it was really a "non-issue." It became a big issue for me, when I decided to go on birth control pills—both for contraceptive reasons and also for relief of severe cramping and pain during menstruation. Birth control coverage was not provided through the insurance plan, as "it was not in keeping with the church's beliefs." Viagra was covered, but not birth control. My doctor was helpful in writing a letter to my agency and health plan, outlining the medical reasons for putting me on Depo Provera. After much run around, I was again denied. It was a frustrating and expensive experience, and if the religious aspect of the agency was "no big deal," why was I denied basic health coverage?

—Theresa, age thirty-one

In the 1990s, mergers between sectarian and nonsectarian hospitals led to the elimination of some or all reproductive services at many hospitals. Catholic hospitals must follow the Ethical and Religious Directives for Catholic Health Care Services, which forbid all reproductive health services that contradict official Catholic teaching, including tubal ligation, vasectomy, abortion, in vitro fertilization, contraceptives, counseling on the use of condoms to prevent HIV/AIDS, and emergency contraception even for rape victims. More than 85 million Americans receive care at hospitals affiliated with the Catholic health care system and most of these patients aren't Catholic and don't share the beliefs of that system. When the sectarian hospital is one of several in town, its ideology is not so great a problem. But when the sectarian provider becomes the majority or only provider, questions must be raised about their ethical responsibility to provide access to the full range of medically and legally acceptable services. Because these hospitals, by and large, all receive our tax dollars, they have a moral obligation to respect the wishes and beliefs of all citizens who receive their services.

The impact of the increased dominance of the Catholic Church in health care is immense:

➤ In New Hampshire, a woman with serious pregnancy complications was forced to leave a Catholic hospital and take an eighty-mile cab ride to find a hospital that would perform the abortion that would save her fertility and maybe her life.

➤ An Alaska woman who delivered her third and last child at a Catholic hospital requested and received a tubal ligation but not a whisper of it appeared in her medical records, where the information might be important for future medical care.

➤ A Gilroy, California, woman tried to schedule a tubal ligation immediately after the birth of her ninth child. But her hospital had been purchased by a Catholic hospital and sterilizations were eliminated. The closest hospital that accepted her medical plan and offered full care was too far away for her to be sure of getting to the maternity ward in time. That left her recovering from childbirth, caring for a large family, and pregnant again before she was able to schedule the surgery.

In some cases, hospitals have maintained reproductive health services through sleight of hand, for example contracting with a separate entity to provide them. But the long-term effectiveness of these compromises is in question. In Austin, Texas, where Catholic Seton Medical Center now runs a city-owned hospital, the original terms of the joint operating agreement allowed tubal ligations to continue. Bishop John McCarthy signed off on the merger, but his policy of allowing tubal ligations was overruled by the Sacred Congregation for the Doctrine of the Faith at the Vatican. Groups like MergerWatch have exposed the immorality and perils of these mergers, and the public has responded.

In Miami, a merger between the Catholic-run Mercy Hospital and the Baptist Health System threatened to severely restrict the availability of abortions in Miami-Dade County. Community activists and physicians took the issue to the public and the Baptist hospitals' board of directors and they won. The stories of these two women had very different outcomes:

 How many women consider that their lives might be saved by legal abortion even if they never have an abortion? In the '50s,

I lived in a small town in the Midwest where the only hospital was Catholic. It was the practice at that time to never lay hands on a woman having a miscarriage unless it could be ascertained that the fetus or embryo was expelled. Medical personnel risked serious legal problems if they were in any way linked with abortion. If you bled to death before they felt free to help you, that was just your bad luck. It happened to a neighbor of mine who left behind a husband and two kids.

—Joyce, late sixties

 Having a child is a choice, and not a choice I wanted to make then, or now, eight years later. I felt no regret or shame in my decision to have an abortion. But I did not want it to happen again, and asked about sterilization. They would not perform such a "permanent procedure" on someone so young (as if having a child isn't a permanent procedure).

—Heather, age thirty

Every minute, a woman dies from barriers to reproductive health care

Sometimes it is easier for us to see these barriers when they are in a global context, but believe me, they exist right here, too. Lack of adequate funding is one of the largest barriers to access in the U.S. and abroad. U.S. commitments to increase funding for international family planning so far are hollow ones. Every minute of every day, a woman dies of mostly preventable pregnancy-related causes in the developing world, the daily equivalent of more than half of the human loss in the World Trade Center attack. One tragedy riveted the attention of the nation and the world. The other continues, day after day, year after year. And the tragedy compounds. When a mother in the developing world dies in childbirth the possibility that her children, up to age ten, will die within two years increases sharply. This is especially true for her daughters.

Guadalupe de la Vega, who is sometimes called the Margaret Sanger of Mexico because she founded a private family planning agency called FEMAP, told me the story of a woman who walked for a day to get to a clinic in Juarez, Mexico. The woman then sat down and asked "How can I get the operation where you tie my legs?" That's how desperate women are to control their fertility, and if it takes a three-hour drive or a daylong walk, they'll do it. But why should they have to?

Around the world, nearly 20 million abortions are performed in unsafe conditions each year, killing more than 80,000 women and filling hospital wards with women suffering debilitating illnesses from unsafe abortion.

Min Min Lama was thirteen when she was raped by her sister-in-law's brother and became pregnant. He was charged but was soon released. When she was several months pregnant, her family arranged for her to have an abortion, which at that time was illegal in her homeland of Nepal. Her sister-in-law reported her to the police. She was arrested and sentenced to a twenty-year term, which she served until the age of fifteen. She was released after successful efforts led by Nepalese activists. (Abortion was legalized in Nepal in September 2002.)

Even the paltry funds that we do send overseas for family planning have restrictions on how they can be used—restrictions that serve only to appease the very vocal anti-choice crowd that helped put George W. Bush in office. One of his first actions was to reinstate the "global gag rule," which denies U.S. family planning funds to nongovernmental organizations overseas if they engage in any activity—even if paid for with their own (non-U.S.) funds—in which the word "abortion" might be mentioned. They can't tell women their options, refer women for abortion to countries where it is legal, or advocate for change in places where it is not. Some groups that are dependent on U.S. funding have interpreted the regulations as precluding them from treating or even referring for treatment women with complications from unsafe abortions.

Peruvian health worker Susana Galdos Silva was so fearful of endangering the family planning funds her group receives from the U.S.

Agency for International Development that she sought and received clearance from a U.S. court before she testified before the Senate Foreign Relations Committee on the impact of the global gag rule in her country. This act illustrated how the global gag rule violates freedom of speech and democratic principles. "When I return to my country tomorrow, I will again be silenced," she said, unable to tell her own legislators what she had told the senators—that 65,000 Peruvian women each year are hospitalized due to complications from unsafe abortions.

In Nepal, the courageous family planning clinic workers who helped Min Min are now in dire financial straits. They have refused to take U.S. funding for family planning with the gag rule attached. The strings attached to the money would keep them from helping girls like Min Min in the future. And because they will have less funding for family planning, the women of Nepal will have more unintended pregnancies and abortions.

Gagged, at home and abroad

The gag rule isn't just an assault on democracy and health care in other countries. It's a spreading stain in the U.S. as well. Domestic gag rules already exist in Colorado and Missouri. Each year we have to fight hard to keep the gag rule off Title X, the backbone of America's family planning program.

Think it through: Let's say you're a Congressman and you oppose abortion. In the U.S. Anywhere. Wouldn't you think that you'd be first in line to vote for more funds for family planning? Or, like Senator Harry Reid, you'd step up to co-sponsor contraceptive equity legislation? In the real world, the cold world of politics, it's too often just the opposite.

Too many anti-choice legislators think they must mollify the extremists who (they think) helped put them in office. And what else do these groups oppose? Contraception, federal funding for family planning, comprehensive, medically accurate sexuality education, insurance coverage for contraceptives, and artificial insemination for infertile couples. Judie Brown, founder of the American Life League, calls emergency contraception "human pesticide."

In the real world, the gift of emergency contraception (a one-time, high dose of the same hormones that are found in birth control pills) is twisted by anti-choice groups from something that prevents a pregnancy from occurring after unprotected sex into an abortifacient, bringing into play all the politics and furor that sadly accompany the abortion issue. As with prescription coverage for contraceptives, the more the public knows about emergency contraception the more it clamors for fairness. Some states and Congress are moving to require emergency room personnel to tell rape victims that emergency contraception is available. Other states now authorize pharmacists to dispense the medication without a physician's prescription, as endorsed by physicians in an article in the *Journal of the American Medical Women's Association*.

In a world with rights but not access, women seeking emergency contraception still are vulnerable to pharmacists who impose their own beliefs on their customers and to hospital emergency rooms, where their options are circumscribed by a set of beliefs that they probably don't share. And 82 percent of the Catholic health system emergency rooms contacted said they did not offer emergency contraception under any circumstances.

When politics trump science, access is denied

In a world where medical decisions bow to politics, the introduction of early nonsurgical abortion (called RU-486 in France and mifepristone in the U.S) nearly stalled, because of fear of anti-choice opposition and of the views of a few executives at the French company Roussel-Uclaf and its German Parent, Hoechst AG. The company placed every possible obstacle in the path of the employees it had assigned to bring the drug to market—limited staff, a surprise withdrawal of the application for approval in France, strict limits on distribution, a stacked vote at a board meeting, and excessively difficult standards for expanding to other countries. When Roussel-Uclaf bowed to protests and withdrew the drug from the market in France, French Health Minster Claude Evin ordered it to reverse its decision, calling mifepristone "the moral property of women."

Finally, pressure from the Clinton administration convinced Roussel-Uclaf, which had refused to market mifepristone in the U.S. because of the political climate, to donate the rights to the drug to the nonprofit Population Council. No established drug manufacturer had the guts to take on the anti-choice lobby—it took a pharmaceutical company formed expressly for the purpose to take mifepristone, through clinical trials and FDA approval, to get the drug to the market in 2000, twelve years after it was approved in France.

The sagas of emergency contraception and mifepristone show how politics can trump science. "Access denied" is the result. The political becomes the personal when millions of U.S. women do not have all of their options available to them.

Denial of services by physical means

But the attitude that one group has the right to impose its beliefs on the rest of us makes politics very personal, day in and day out, for the people who work at reproductive health clinics and for the women who visit the clinics seeking to plan their families:

 I especially resented having to push past clinic protestors just to see my doctor (for treatment of pre-cancerous cells). How do they know who is having an abortion? Does it make sense to block women from clinics where they can get birth control?
—Tracy, age twenty-nine

And how many frightened young women just turn around and go home access denied by fear of harassment? We'll never know exactly. But this I do know. Protesters almost never—*never*—deter a woman seeking abortion. That decision, once made, is urgent, and every minute is critical. Getting birth control or other health care is merely important and therefore more easily deferred when a woman doesn't want to walk a gauntlet of protestors. How many unintended pregnancies and abortions have been caused by the very people whose mission it is to eliminate abortion all together?

Chapter Eleven
Whose conscience counts?

 I made my choice for the love of life.

—Sharon, fifty-four

There are three exceptions I have seen anti-choice people make with regularity: Rape, incest, and "me."

So I watched with great interest the debate over whether President George W. Bush would approve federal funding for research using stem cells from embryos. Many lawmakers who say they believe the fetus holds equal status with or primacy over the woman made an exception: here, the embryo could be subordinated to the needs of actual people—in this case, their own needs or the needs of the people they love.

Such hypocrisy permeates the anti-choice position on reproductive self-determination. Representative Bob Barr of Georgia once told me and several other pro-choice leaders the following during a congressional hearing: "I think the four of you," he scolded us, "have become very hardened, very cold, and very callous . . . you really have developed, I'm sad to say, a moral blind spot."

We had testified that Congress should not practice medicine and that reproductive health decisions should be made by women with their families and physicians, not by government. In my testimony, I told the stories of several women and their experiences with tragic and catastrophic pregnancies that had necessitated wrenching choices. My testimony concluded with the following:

 This bill trivializes women who must make difficult decisions under circumstances that, quite frankly, would soundly defeat many of us here today. In the quarter century since *Roe v. Wade*, American women have not had a moment's rest—not from legislative attempts to restrict their rights, not from violent protesters willing to use any means to interfere with their private and personal decisions. I have personally worked to promote and protect women's health for all those years, and I am still amazed at those who would say to a woman, "We are not your doctors, we are not your family, but we are going to tell you what to do."

Eli's coming, do anti-choice politicians care?

It was more than annoying to me that I had received the "request" to appear at this hearing while I was in Arizona awaiting the birth of a grandchild. I wanted to be there with my daughter Linda for Eli's lovingly awaited birth. The anti-choice senators and representatives on the two judiciary committees never did quite grasp the irony of their demand that I drop everything and rush back to appear before them in Washington to defend a woman's right to abortion at this particular moment.

On the plane back to Arizona from Washington, I thought long and hard about who has the moral blind spot and whose conscience counts in these difficult childbearing decisions.

When it comes to childbearing, it is the very fortunate among us who have not wrestled with the kind of gut-wrenching life choices that test who we are at the core. If we're lucky, we never have to sit in a dimly lit hospital room and listen to a physician lay out an array of grim scenarios, each more heartbreaking than the last. But not every woman is so lucky. As I think back to the hearing room, I do not recall any reflection in those lawmakers' eyes of the women whose lives and health are in the balance. In their moral prism, there was only room for the fetus.

Respect for women is still not there. Their latest juggernaut aimed at recriminalizing abortion is to pass laws and policies that would give the fetus status separate from and greater than that of the woman. These lawmakers are intent on redefining the fetus so that it has primacy, by making the fetus, not the pregnant woman, eligible for prenatal care under the State Child Health Insurance Program. And they're creating criminal penalties for harming the fetus, separate from penalties for harming the pregnant woman. These measures make the plot of Margaret Atwood's *The Handmaid's Tale* seem all too plausible. Women as mere vessels for reproduction may sound like speculative fiction, but we had better stop this emerging legislative strategy now or life may well soon imitate art.

Who has a conscience?

The same holds true for legislation that allows health care professionals to deny, without penalty, medically accepted reproductive health services to women who want them, because of the legislators' personal or religious beliefs. Our legislators are telling us whose conscience counts and it's not mine, and it's probably not yours, either.

It is not an act of conscience to refuse to provide family planning and abortion. It is an act of discrimination. Sometimes it is an act of medical malpractice. Always it is a refusal to provide legal and medically appropriate options to a patient whose conscience should be considered above others. And it assumes, arrogantly, that those hospitals, insurance plans, and medical personnel who do provide family planning and abortion services have no consciences. As if the doctors who place a woman's health first have no consciences. As if the women who receive such care have no consciences. As if their consciences just don't count.

I wonder what the Bob Barrs of the world really want when they oppose abortion; when they question the moral integrity of the women who have to make, and live with, these decisions. Why are they so obsessed with other peoples' sex lives? They can't argue they want improved lives for women and children; legislators who want to deny women's right to choose abortion do little to help women prevent pregnancy in the first place or to raise the children they do have. In fact, a 1991 Catholics for a Free Choice study found that members of Congress who oppose abortion are more likely to vote against social programs that benefit women, children, and families.

Claremont Graduate University political science professor Jean Schroedel surveyed state policies. She found that the strongest prochoice states spend more per child on foster care, stipends for foster parents who adopt special needs children, and funding for poor women with dependent children than do states with the most stringent anti-abortion laws. States with the most onerous laws limiting abortion spent the least on needy children. Though she had not been an activist before this, Schroedel said her findings, published in 1999, were so striking that she promptly joined several pro-choice organizations. "Pro-life states make it difficult for women to have abortions, but they do not help these women provide for the children once born," she said.

Exposing the anti-choice moral blind spot

What is morally wrong with women taking responsibility for their own lives? What is morally wrong with women making moral choices about childbearing? And what gives members of Congress or anyone the right to judge them? Just whose moral blind spot have we exposed? Whose conscience counts?

And what about Bob Barr's own moral blind spot? How can someone who advocates tirelessly for abortion to be illegal again rationalize paying for his second wife's abortion? We've all seen the check he wrote displayed on national television. How can someone who feels he holds the moral high ground justify the fact that at the same time, he was apparently involved with the woman who became his third wife?

Wait—I know. It's one of the three exceptions. "It's me." Here are two women who saw the light:

 I knew what I had to do before I made the decision. I was going through a rough time and I couldn't support myself and my first child. I had always been pro life, quietly, until it was my problem. I have to say, I am a lot better off now. I would rather have not had to have an abortion, but I don't regret it. I believe that everyone has the right to their own opinion. But I prefer that they keep their rosaries out of my ovaries. The way I look at it is, if you don't think it is right to have an abortion, don't.

—Ceil, age thirty-two

 We were young, we made a mistake, and I had an abortion. It almost hurts to say that word, but I can say it. It took time for my mind and heart to heal and they have. I am a responsible person who decided a situation was not right for me. I could not bear the emotional, mental, or financial responsibility of a child. Oh, did I mention that previous to this experience I was anti-choice. One can never have true feelings about pregnancy until they are there.

—Mariah, age twenty-two

I met Cyprian Awiti, who runs the Marie Stopes clinics in Kenya, while on a visit to see family planning programs there. He shines the light on the hypocrisy with this question: "Who is more the murderer? The woman who has an abortion or the person who refuses to provide her a safe abortion and she dies?"

Making choices for the love of life

Sharon is the woman whose phrase "I made my choice for the love of life" introduces this chapter. She wrote to tell me the full context of her life affirming choice:

 I was a married United Methodist Minister with a child and a five-month-old infant when the Supreme Court handed down *Roe v. Wade*. Five days later, I found out I was pregnant—in spite of my IUD. I was physically and emotionally exhausted and already felt I couldn't handle my responsibilities to my family and my ministry. My doctor discussed all my options, including abortion. I went home and, with my husband and in the light of our own faith tradition, we decided we could not accept the risks to the quality of life for our existing family that adding to it would entail. Even today, thirty years later, I feel relief and a sense of having made the right—the moral—choice. I believed then and I believe now that as a Christian, I needed to do what was life-enhancing. I made my choice for the love of life.

—Sylvia, age fifty-four

And who has the right to decide that safe reproductive health services will not be available in a community? Increasingly, those decisions are made by elderly, celibate men. I wonder if they have any way of understanding what it is like for a woman to bear a child, recover from the birth, care for that child, and then schedule a second medical procedure from which she also will have to recover—at a different, less convenient or less familiar facility. Simply because these men, who don't even try to imagine walking in another person's shoes, deny her the right to end her fertility. These men are so different from that kindly priest who introduced me and so many of the women in his parish to Planned Parenthood because he was able to empathize with their difficulties. People have differing beliefs. That's entirely legitimate. It's the arrogance of placing the validity of your beliefs over mine in such a personal matter that creates acrimony and endless debate.

Again, Reverend J. Philip Wogaman:

 How difficult [anti-choice fanatics] can be! Sometimes I think the supreme test of love is whether we can love people who don't love us—just as the final mark of tolerance is to be able to tolerate the intolerant. Certainly it does not mean to give in to their wishes and allow them to suffocate the right to choose.

Still, we cannot allow hate-filled rhetoric and mean-spirited acts to corrupt our own spirits with hate. It helps to understand where much of this is coming from. It helps to see that the seed-bed of fanaticism is spiritual insecurity. Our response can be a bit more like what some of the people in my church did one day when we were being picketed by a religious hate group. It was an extremely cold day, and our people greeted the demonstrators outside with hot chocolate and donuts.

A few days after the congressional hearing, I appeared on a television show to debate a congressman who is virulently opposed to abortion. Throughout the program, my gaze kept drifting toward a young female makeup artist. She stayed on the set throughout the taping and watched the proceedings with a stricken look. Afterward, she told me that this was her first day back at work after having an abortion. Her wanted pregnancy, you see, had gone terribly, tragically wrong. "Don't these politicians understand?" she said. "This is about women's health."

I wish she could have posed the question to the congressman, but I suppose he hadn't seen her. Something must have blocked his view.

The conscience of a pro-choicer

➤ We believe in the right to sexual and reproductive self-determination that is non-coercive, non-exploitive, and responsible.

➤ We believe that the free and joyous expression of one's own sexuality is central to being fully human.

➤ We believe in trusting individuals and providing them with the information they need to make well-informed decisions about sexuality, family planning, and childbearing.

➤ We believe that women should have an equal place at life's table, and be respected as moral decision makers.

➤ We believe that children flourish best in families and communities where they are nurtured, honored and loved.

➤ We believe in passion—for change, for justice, for easing the plight of others, for caring, for living our convictions, and for confronting inhumane acts.

➤ We believe in action—to make things happen and to improve people's lives and circumstances.

➤ We believe in inclusion and diversity—and the power and knowledge they confer.

➤ We believe the future is global and that we are part of a global movement.

➤ We believe in the urgency of creating a sustainable world and living in peace with our planet.

➤ We believe in leadership based upon collaboration rather than hierarchy.

➤ We believe in acting courageously, especially as allies with those who have little or no voice and little or no power.

➤ We believe that every right is tied to responsibility and that the fulfillment of responsibility is itself a source of joy.

—Statement of Beliefs,
adopted by Planned Parenthood Federation
of America membership, March 2001.

Chapter Twelve
Murder in the name of life

When you multiply the intolerance and the ideological fanaticism of a Bob Barr or a Jerry Falwell by the others who share their views, and you take their assumed moral righteousness to its logical conclusion, you can predict tragedy.

 Three months after [a counselor in Brookline helped me], a man walked into that clinic and opened fire, killing my counselor. What had she done to deserve that? She had helped a broken little girl make the biggest decision of her life. She had supported me when the man responsible was missing. She helped prepare me to be the mother I will become. And now she's gone.

—Alexis, age twenty-five

Righteous wrongs

The streets of New York, normally a cacophony of sound, were eerily still that Wednesday morning. No traffic. No hot dog or pretzel vendors. No taxis. No dog walkers. No fashionable commuters, rushing along in tennis shoes. As I walked, my view down Sixth Avenue from miles north of the World Trade Center was unobstructed. What was most noticeable was what you knew wasn't there anymore. In its place, white and gray smoke billowed in clouds that would have been beautiful if they hadn't represented something horrible beyond imagining. It was September 12, 2001, the day after everything changed forever. That morning, the people of the United States of America and the world awoke to a reality that we finally, cruelly, horribly, were forced to acknowledge, the reality that people who hate are capable of catastrophic acts of terror with thousands of innocents as their victims. We are all vulnerable.

Commentators said we shouldn't be so surprised. The rhetoric and the threats had assaulted us for years. Criticism on the world stage. Foreign leaders denouncing the U.S. Fringe groups emerging from the heat of the rhetoric. Then action. Barracks bombed. Airliners destroyed in midflight. Embassies bombed. One of our military warships the target of suicide bombers. A plot to disrupt millennium celebrations.

As the hate fed the violence and both were fed by fear, we listened, watched, and worried, but felt secure in the midst of a pluralistic society in which bloodshed over differing views was incomprehensible to most Americans. Many of the perpetrators of the acts against the U.S., and all of the masterminds, faded into safe harbors provided by those who despise our way of life, who would substitute their narrow view of the world for our tolerance for differences; their rigid philosophies for our glorious independence.

We reacted, each time, to the individual incidents. But how could we assimilate into our view of the world the extent of the horror that really was out there? How could we believe that what we viewed as a clash of cultures or ideologies or religions could escalate into this kind of terrorism?

The ugly face of terrorism

My heart hurt for the loss of life that brought grief to thousands and for what each individual, no matter how far removed from the tragedy, had lost: the feeling of safety and security in our own land. But while these feelings of insecurity, of imminent threat, were new to most Americans, they have long been a way of life for me and the thousands of men and women who provide reproductive health care. My colleagues and I know far too much about the ugly face of terrorism. Sadly, this is a bond we now share with the nation.

Tom Webber tells us how it got to be that way:

 As the CEO of a large, two-state Planned Parenthood affiliate for the better part of three decades, I had a front-line position to not simply observe, but to experience, the anti-abortion movement. The violence in Minnesota started in 1976. We had two fires in 1977 alone. We had become accustomed to the high flourish of anti-choice rhetoric. But we, the pro-choice people, had a disbelief and an unwillingness to look at what happens when the social climate becomes that full of hatred. The outcome—of great violence—was inevitable, but nobody wanted to acknowledge it. Basically nobody could believe what was happening.

I had a seat to experience the threats to the daughter of a Board member—a young girl who found a note in her school locker threatening to do her harm if her mother did not leave her position on the Planned Parenthood Board of Directors. The school could not guarantee the safety of that young girl, and she ultimately was removed from school and moved to another city when her mother refused to resign her Board position.

I experienced this component of the anti-abortion movement up close and personal when I found a note in my home mailbox. It was a rather crude note. It claimed to know where our two daughters went to school, and it threatened to place them in harm's way. I tried to calm my wife all the while struggling to control the fear and the rage within. The following morning, I telephoned the local police department only to find that my wife was already there speaking with one of the command officers. We lived with a police car outside our door until the threat was deemed to have passed. Never again did either of our daughters take the bus to school. They did not walk nor ride their bikes. Either their mother or I took them every day until they successfully graduated.

The devolution to violence

When anti-choice groups first moved from rhetoric to picketing to mass demonstrations, the prevailing pro-choice attitude was not to dignify them with a reaction. And why should we? We had the high ground. What we were doing was legal, it was morally and socially laudable for its positive impact on women and their families, it was supported by many diverse faiths and by a majority of the American people, and it was critically important to women's lives. We were the establishment. They were just expressing their differing views, and they had a right to do so. We respected their right to hold contrary ideas and even take to the streets in support of them; we tolerated their protests as part of the process, and we discounted the words of hate that emerged from their most extreme fringe and began to pollute the social climate.

But pickets and protests became blockades and bombs. Petty vandalism, broken windows, and glued locks became routine. The people opposed to a woman's right to make her own childbearing decisions inexorably climbed the steps toward violence.

My own first experience with a clinic invasion was when a group of a dozen or so people, including several children who inexplicably wore knitted woolen toboggan hats in the middle of summer, swarmed into our downtown Phoenix facility. They had arrived from California in an old yellow school bus. They terrorized people in the waiting room. An alert staff quickly sealed off the examining rooms. Two of the protesters chained themselves to a desk. About this time, the local television station's cameras arrived, invited by the protestors to witness this theatrical performance. The police came, the chains were sawed, and the protesters were removed in wheelchairs borrowed from the nearby hospital, all of this on camera. I stepped out of a staff meeting to give my statement to the reporters. Whew, that's over, we thought. But it had just begun.

The demonstrators went from Operation Rescue to their self-described Year of Pain and Fear. Since one of the key organizers of this nationwide onslaught was John Jakubczyk of Phoenix, I got special attention. Every day, my staff and I drove through hordes of picketers brandishing disgusting signs, often hurling epithets at us by name. Every day, far worse, women coming to our clinics—including those coming for birth control or Pap smears—had to walk through demonstrators who called themselves "sidewalk counselors." I suppose some of the birth control clients turned away, intimidated by the spectacle. But the women seeking abortions came anyway, even though the medical evidence showed that they experienced elevated blood pressure and greater physical pain.

Joseph Feldman, who runs the clinic in Phoenix, still sees this every day:

 A Vietnamese couple came to our abortion program because the wife was pregnant, a wanted pregnancy, but there were several fetal anomalies, including a condition in which there is fetal kidney failure and another in which amniotic fluid is too scarce. The wife spoke no English. Her husband spoke broken English. "My English . . . stuck," he said. The husband displayed nothing but love and concern for his wife. He had many questions. Did his case of herpes cause the fetal defects? Why was his baby sick? Why were the picketers yelling at him? "They say I kill my baby," he told the nurse-midwife, Joanne, "but I ask them, 'You fix my baby?' and they say they cannot. Why they yell like that?"

How does one explain the politics and cultural conflict surrounding abortion to a loving Vietnamese husband? On the morning of the surgery, the husband explained that "after you take the baby out, I pour water over the baby." So, after the surgery, in a private room, Joanne and I showed him the fetal remains in a plastic container. I brought him some water, and he poured a few drops over the remains. The three of us stood in silence for a moment, each lost in our own thoughts. Then the husband signaled that he was done, and I removed the remains, his son, and he went to sit in the lobby and wait for his wife to recover. A moment later, Joanne and I met in the hall and hugged each other, each impressed by the sacred moment we had shared with this man. The picketers yell at us each morning, or pray for us, or whatever they do . . . but inside the clinic, we know we are doing God's work.

That's how it feels inside the clinic. So not surprisingly, my first response to the harassment by anti-choice demonstrators was to take solace in the satisfaction of helping people and to ignore those who trespassed against us. And the response of my pro-choice colleagues was similar. We occasionally held genteel, pro-choice gatherings, while nearby, protestors loudly circled the offices of doctors who performed abortions. One day my husband, Alex, had had enough. He took the podium and exhorted the crowd to march, and he led us to the doctor's office to bear witness in his defense. Action made us feel better, but did little to stem the tide.

Alex's reaction was a rare one. It is inherently difficult for pro-choice people who value tolerance and diversity to assert their passion in a confrontational way. Like most Americans, who are open and tolerant, we didn't realize that in the end, our adversaries would neither respect nor tolerate our rights to our own beliefs, and that in the end, much of the pro-choice majority and especially those who are opinion leaders—by their silence and their incredulity—were complicit with the extremists that had created this toxic social climate. In the end, this formidable enemy would neither respect nor tolerate our very existence, our right to life. The inevitable result was murder.

No other side to murder

I can't think of another instance, ever, where Americans exercising their legal rights have had to undergo such harassment for so long with so little support from so much of law enforcement. Civil rights activists in the 1960s received similar treatment as they attempted to change the law. Imagine if you had to endure that kind of gauntlet to attend your chosen house of worship, or express your views at a routine city council meeting.

The media bear special culpability. If Planned Parenthood opened a new health center where thousands of women could get low cost gynecological care and birth control, they paid no attention. If a single picketer showed up with a gruesome sign at this new health center, the cameras were there for the photo opportunity. Sometimes we joked that we should hire a few picketers just so we could get some free advertising.

But even worse is the media's polarization of the issues by always insisting on presenting the "other side"—even when the topic is as innocuous as the introduction of a new birth control method or a community educational program for parents. Even when there has been a murder. They corrupt our very language when they accept the term "pro-life" for people who threaten the lives of others. I believe it is much more pro-life to be pro-choice, to value the fullness and richness of human life, and to encompass all views on this complex moral issue. In contrast, the anti-choice position respects no views but its own.

After Dr. Barnett Slepian was murdered by a sniper while talking with his sons in the kitchen of his home in Buffalo, New York, I appeared on CNN's *Talk Back Live* with Bobbie Batista. The producer had assured me that I would be appearing alone to talk with Bobbie and the audience about the murder and its implications. Lo and behold, as the camera started rolling—I was appearing from a remote studio—Bobbie introduced a woman from National Right to Life representing the "other side."

This was the first and only time I lambasted an interviewer on live TV. "The other side? There is no other side to murder," I said.

Then, with a straight face, a perfectly normal looking woman in a polka-dot dress told America that she understood how the murderer could have become so frustrated at his inability to outlaw abortion that he murdered another human being.

Because I have made defending women's health and women's reproductive choices my life's work, my family and I have been forced to get used to certain things. I'm accustomed to personal epithets and ugly threats from those who claim to own all enlightenment and morality. They just reinforce my commitment to my cause. I'm used to rings of picketers forming a welcome wagon at our new home. ("Gloria Feldt is a rich, classy murderer" one sign said.) This incivility provided me with the opportunity to be quickly welcomed also by my new neighbors, who brought gifts and words of support.

I'm used to being told to travel with a security guard, and not to work in a bright, open office because I'd be an all-too-easy target for violence. Bombs have been thrown inside our offices. Less harmful but quite unappealing were the chicken livers thrown onto our doors. Some providers experienced butyric acid attacks that filled the building with putrid-smelling chemicals.

Appeasing the crocodile

In some cities, local police were responsive and helpful from the beginning. But reaction to the escalating anti-choice onslaught from most law enforcement at all levels could, at best, be described as complacent. They seemed to rather enjoy the spectacle at first. They lost track of who was the perpetrator and who was the victim. When I warned the Phoenix chief of police about potentially violent protests, he said, point-blank, "Close the clinic that day." That, of course, is the exact opposite of the right response. We weren't doing anything wrong, but the blockaders certainly were. I went over his head to the mayor and the tune changed.

When I received a series of death threats on my home phone in neo-Nazi language, the police provided no help until I prevailed on a friend on the force to take charge. But the responsible parties were never found. It took years of meeting with law enforcement representatives, and a federal law called the Freedom of Access to Clinic Entrances Act, before we began to receive appropriate protection for our facilities and our personnel.

Anthrax threats are not new to us—before September 11, Planned Parenthood offices had received more than sixty of them, starting in 1998. When the subsequent rash of 500 anthrax threats began arriving at women's reproductive health providers across the country, our staffs already were opening the mail with masks and gloves. They followed our long-established protocols, protocols so good that they were adapted by the FBI for their own use. Fortunately, none of the letters contained actual anthrax, but they nevertheless were fearsome vessels of terrorism.

After intense efforts on our part, the U.S. Department of Justice finally classified these kinds of attacks as hate crimes. After September 11, that classification was quickly upgraded to domestic terrorism. And it became clear to the American people that the terrorists who target women's clinics are a threat to our democracy that law enforcement should take seriously.

Today, Web sites operated by anti-choice extremists track doctors and others involved in providing abortion services. Photos, home addresses, and other personal information are posted on hit lists. Web cameras broadcast images of women entering clinics, and private medical records have even been stolen and posted on line. The purveyors of these websites like to call what they are doing "free speech." I know it to be a true threat, and I think any reasonable person would percieve it that way, too.

Only minutes after Dr. Slepian was killed, a line was drawn through his name on one such Web site. Since President Bush announced that limited stem cell research should go forward, his name has been added to the Web site's hit list. That's how extreme these people are.

U.S. Attorney General John Ashcroft at first declined to send federal marshals to protect a targeted doctor during mass protests in Wichita, Kansas, in August 2001 until a news conference held by pro-choice organizations in Washington, DC, created enough pressure to force him to act. Mind you, the last time this kind of mass protest was held in Wichita, the same doctor was shot and wounded. Mind you also that Mr. Ashcroft had just addressed a conference on domestic terrorism, declaring his intent to make eradicating it a priority.

Those federal marshals were a big help in letting the Wichita demonstrators know they had to remain peaceful this time. But what made an even greater difference was the community support and preparedness, especially the coalition of clergy from many faiths, organized by the Religious Coalition for Reproductive Choice, in support of the doctor, civility, and a woman's right to choose. They sent a clear signal that violence would not be accommodated in Wichita.

I have learned that accommodating extremists just leads to more extremism. It is folly to appease terrorists of any kind. As Winston Churchill put it, "An appeaser is someone who feeds the crocodile hoping it will eat him last."

From Tom Webber:

 Unfortunately, the anti-choice movement has within its core a disquieting and dangerous component of extremists—and worse—zealots. It is this component that has too often framed the public discourse through its actions of high theater, flamboyance, and abject violation of law and insult upon human dignity. These zealots thought they had ultimate truth. They believed there were evil ogres inside the clinic building. And they used other inflammatory rhetoric to create that climate in which the violence would become inevitable.

I don't care who lit the match, the anti-choice movement was responsible for creating the climate that burned the Minnesota clinic to the ground on Ash Wednesday 1977.

I experienced this component when an escapee of a mental treatment facility gained access to my office by posing as a reporter from a religious newspaper wishing to do an interview. After accusing me of "murdering Jesus Christ," he calmly stated that Christ had commanded him to murder me. And he nearly did. Had the physical assault not occurred at my place of employment, I am convinced the damages would have been far worse. When colleagues came to my aid, we found the pockets of the man to be filled with the anti-abortion literature passed out by extremist abortion opponents. I could not comprehend then, nor can I now, how in the name of whatever they hold as holy, the leadership of the anti-abortion movement failed to grasp that they had set the climate for the extremists within their movement.

The "antis" not only hate abortion and those who provide that care, but also family planning programs. I have never found the anti-abortion movement to support family planning programs at state or federal levels. To the contrary, family planning programs became just one more vehicle for them to use to promote their opposition to abortion. In retrospect, we should have acted more strongly and sooner. It was in effect permitted to go on. Nobody was ever caught. If it had been a synagogue or a black church or the Girl Scouts or anybody else, this kind of violence would never have been tolerated.

A tale of extraordinary courage

Nicki Nichols Gamble spent decades as president of Planned Parenthood League of Massachusetts and describes a similar devolution to violence:

 Physicians were targeted. One physician's home was picketed. She had small children. There was enormous anxiety and fear that was created for her because of this. There was a constant sense that somebody close was not far from violence.

The climate that is created when the moral choices of women are subordinated, when their lives and health are ignored in favor of the potential life of the fetus, is a climate of hate that fosters a climate of violence. For hate and violence grow best in an atmosphere that is devoid of respect for people with differing views. I recall clearly the day I was on the phone with June Barrett, who with her husband had been an escort for women trying to get through the protestors at a Pensacola, Florida, clinic. June's husband was murdered as was the doctor they had been escorting. I was making arrangements for her to come to Phoenix to speak about her experiences when a call came in from a friend whose granddaughter volunteered at Nicki's Brookline, Massachusetts, clinic. She had called to tell me her grandmother was safe. Not everyone at the clinic was so lucky.

Nicki remembers:

 There had been a six-year backdrop of unbelievable Operation Rescue demonstrations. I would wake up in the middle of the night on Friday nights asking myself, "How long can I personally stand to be part of this?" The anxiety, the worry, the sense of responsibility were just overwhelming. Our concerns were elevated and we worked on strategies to protect people as they came and went from their clinics. Nevertheless, John Salvi's actions were like an earthquake, a watershed. As much as we had seen, it was a shock. Having someone walk into your facility in broad daylight and kill one and injure three and then go down the street and kill another person was simply beyond imagining. Shannon Lowney's body was on the floor with a sheet over it when I arrived at the clinic. It lay there for hours while the police did their work. It was a bright beautiful sunny day with a cold blue sky. Inside we were in shock. We were traumatized. Every year on the anniversary there are memorial services. It will be with me the rest of my life.

The hate feeds the violence and both are fed by fear. Our adversaries are terrified of us because they fear that what we do changes the roles of women and elevates women's status, and they think this will change their world irrevocably. They are, of course, right about that. They can clearly see how today's world has been shaped by the reproductive rights movement—and they don't like it one bit. That part I can understand. I am not able to grasp why they think that gives them the right to attack violently those with whom they disagree.

Here's Nicki again:

 What's different about violence against reproductive health care is that it is not random. We are specifically targeted. It is targeted toward people who are serving women primarily. It is deep-seated, religious, and misogynistic antipathy toward us that encourages people to want to blow us up and kill us. It is fueled by a point of view that is never going to go away. We will never *not* have serious enemies because they have particular animosity toward sexuality, toward equality for women and children, they have a virulent misogyny and sometimes serious psychological problems among some of them. There is a political strain of animosity that comes out of the worst hypocrisy I've ever felt. Many politicians who are anti-choice, anti-family planning, and anti-sex education lead reprehensible lives. And yet they use this issue for their own ends.

Learning about sexuality and childbearing is as important as learning to read and write. It's a key foundational skill. But these people want to be in charge of everybody else's decisions. They don't want uppity women speaking up to them. They want their children to be their property, not to grow and develop. They are controlling, ideological, and have a hostile mentality. They want to call the shots rather than enabling people to grow themselves. In contrast, my husband Dick wants me to be all that I can be. It's such a difference.

A difference with a distinction between pro- and anti-choice positions

It's not just a difference. It's two entirely different worldviews. The question then becomes, do those who oppose us have the right to force us to live according to their rules, and their rules alone? The answer, in a democracy, is no. But I do expect them to respect my positions as I have respected theirs. As one patient put it:

 Unlike the anti-choice groups, God is all-understanding.
—Janice, age thirty-four

A fundamental difference between the pro-choice and anti-choice positions is that the pro-choice position allows for and respects the anti-choice position. No one has to have an abortion regardless of what society thinks about that person's appropriateness as a parent. The pro-choice position defends your right not to choose abortion. Suffice it to say that it would never occur to me to try to pressure an anti-choice doctor to perform abortions by picketing his home and vilifying him because he wouldn't change his stripes.

Here's a real-life experience that I witnessed. A fourteen-year-old made an appointment for an abortion. She already had a five-month-old baby. Both she and the baby lived with her mother; all were on welfare. The mother was absolutely convinced that abortion was the best course of action. Neither the mother nor the daughter was willing to consider adoption though we had discussed it with them. The fourteen-year-old had been counseled about her options, had evidenced an ability to understand them, and had made the decision to have an abortion after an informed consent process. But when she came in for the procedure, she changed her mind. Her mother was furious with us for not persuading her to have an abortion. Objectively, I can say that this young woman made a choice that ultimately may not have been in her best interest nor that of society and almost certainly not that of her five-month-old. But it was her informed decision and she will have to live with it.

When people hold differing views about such deeply personal matters, in a democracy, the individual—not the government, and certainly not the person who differs from you—has the right and responsibility to decide. And that is not an abdication of moral values. It is an affirmation of some of the highest moral values of a pluralistic democracy: freedom, respect, personal integrity.

As Tom Webber said to me:

 As a social fabric, we must have the ability to vigorously hold different views on matters of substance. We must do more than tolerate our differences. We must celebrate and protect them. We cannot ever cease to acknowledge the righteousness of our differences and the value of their worth. The anti-abortion movement, or at least some components of it, fails miserably in this regard.

Unfortunately, neither our founding fathers nor our anti-choice adversaries today, nor for that matter, the Taliban, heeded Abigail Adams' admonition to "remember the ladies." But futurist Watts Wacker, who wrote to tell me why he and his wife escort patients every

Saturday, and have done so for ten years, does remember why it is so important for citizens to act on their pro-choice convictions. He says, "The fastest route to self-esteem is to stand up for what you believe." He puts his convictions into action every week, not by destroying or threatening those with whom he disagrees but by helping those who need him:

 Perhaps the most thought provoking event, for me, was the first time I opened the car door to assist the doctor from the passenger side of his "delivery" car and upon extending my arm to him realized that he was wearing a bulletproof vest... and I was not!! Soon my wife Betsy and I realized that we should never stand next to each other while we escort. But if I really had to come down to one reason why I escort, it can be told in what has sadly become virtually the same story for every client of our clinic. The client and a partner arrive. They park their car on a public street and walk on a public sidewalk to the clinic. They immediately are confronted with protesters who demand answers to questions like . . . "Are you here to murder your child?"

The patient is presented with both escorts and protesters. Escorts ask if they would like assistance in reaching the building. Protestors assume that they have a right to ask, and have you answer their questions . . . as well as to insist on giving you their literature. In all of my experience, every single incident, if a client merely says, "Would you please leave me alone," I have never seen a protester recede. Not once have they acknowledged the client's rights to believe in something that they do not. If I could believe that a client could look at a protester and say, "Please, please leave me alone. No thank you for your literature," and the protesters would walk away, then, and only then do I think I could stop escorting.

Life lessons learned in the crucible

We in the reproductive health and rights movement can teach some life lessons to the rest of America as we all struggle to heal and move forward from the terrorist attacks of September 11.

First, it is possible to recover from such a tragedy and keep the integrity of mission and purpose intact; indeed, to recover with our mission and purpose even stronger. I never cease to be humbled and awed by the thousands of people like Tom and Nicki and June Barrett and Shannon Lowney's family, who even as they mourned, recommitted themselves to securing simple justice for women.

Second, it is possible to balance absolute commitment to personal freedom with an equally absolute commitment to the safety of our people. We know our purpose, assess our risks, and implement protocols accordingly, from bulletproof glass to video cameras to analyzing telephoned bomb threats. Reproductive health care providers have developed amazingly effective ways to be safe from terrorism and violence while creating a welcoming place for their patients, staffs, and volunteers. Many spend huge sums of money to make this safety as invisible as possible. But my favorite example is a clinic that installed a noisy leaf blower on a patch of grassy yard facing the sidewalk where particularly loud and aggressive picketers regularly congregate. They named it "Wooly Bully," and attached a boombox to play the song of the same name at full volume during all picketing sessions. You can't help but laugh, and that reduces the tension.

Third, the best way to achieve that balance between safety and freedom is for leaders in the community—and all the rest of us—to stand together courageously against the violence, regardless of their stance on abortion. This alone can create the social climate in which violence is extinguished because it simply never gets any oxygen. That's what happened in Wichita the second time it was targeted, and it worked. The protestors got their freedom of speech, but no one was hurt and women had access to the care they wanted.

Finally, it is important to restore normality as soon as possible, to go back to business as usual, for in so doing, we bear witness to the simple fact that terrorists cannot deter us from our mission, cannot destroy our way of life or sway us from our principles. All terrorists are joined at the head. Their aim is to create mass hysteria and stop us from doing our work. When they do deter us, they have won. Action is the best antidote to the powerless feeling that comes after an attack, and remaining on course is our best revenge against terrorism. That's why our clinics remained open or reopened as soon as law enforcement and public health officials permitted it after the anthrax threats, and why to the best of our knowledge not one patient went unserved. This courage and commitment is what gives people hope for the future.

As I write in 2002, National Guard reservists guard our airports as the passengers who have returned to the skies snake through long security lines. While the terrorist attack has united our country in grim determination, this new world remains one of vulnerability and trepidation unthinkable a few months ago.

The Reverend Pat Robertson has left his position as head of the Christian Coalition—soon after he and Jerry Falwell blamed the World Trade Center attack on, basically, everyone who disagrees with them—pagans, feminists, gays and lesbians, "abortionists," and the ACLU. "God will not be mocked," they say, seemingly forgetting that many people even they would consider good Christians were killed—and one of the heroes who diverted the fourth plane was a gay man. They seemingly do not realize that Osama bin Laden, too, vilified a people with whom he disagreed.

And the connection between the terrorists of the World Trade Center and the domestic terrorists that stalk reproductive health care workers has come full circle. The U.S. Marshal's Service has arrested an escaped felon, Clayton Lee Waagner, whose anti-abortion crusade, fueled by firearms, bombs, and stolen vehicles, has been familiar to law enforcement officials for some time. At his previous trial in December of 2000, he testified that he'd been stockpiling weapons to use against doctors who provided abortions because God has asked him to "be my warrior." According to a posting on the Army of God Web site, he has since broadened his scope because "I have discovered the hard way just how difficult these 'doctors' are to get to. I'm going after everyone else. It doesn't matter to me if you're a nurse, receptionist, bookkeeper or a janitor, if you work for the murderous abortionist, I'm going to kill you. We'll get this terrorism thing started in earnest." Here's the final straw. Clayton Lee Waagner has also claimed credit for piggybacking on our national tragedy of fear and death, and sending out the five hundred anthrax threats to reproductive health clinics.

How dare they call themselves "pro-life?" How can anyone think this is "pro-life?" Waagner has earned a lifetime prison sentence. The dedication of the reproductive health care workers and supporters who put their lives on the line ought to earn them a Nobel Peace Prize. I personally feel profoundly honored to be in their company and to speak for this great cause.

We can succeed in fighting terrorism, foreign and domestic, if we heed what Dee Hock, the creator of the Visa card concept that revolutionized commerce globally, says about making change: "First they laugh at you, then they fight you, and then you win." We can succeed if we approach change strengthened by the very thing the terrorists hate: our diversity, our tolerance for each other, and our intolerance of intolerance.

Seeing the diversity of New York back on the streets just weeks after the attack was a pleasure for the senses. Think about it: Cantor Fitzgerald, the firm that sustained the greatest number of losses, has diversity written all over its name. What could be more American? At St. Patrick's Cathedral, where a funeral for a victim of the September 11 attacks was about to begin, men with green ribbons and shamrocks greeted each other outside. The strains of a bagpipe playing "Amazing Grace" could be heard coming from within the church. As I rounded the corner, the bagpiper—a woman—walked out of the church's front door.

I think to myself: they are right, those terrorists who gave their lives in an attempt to destroy America and our symbols of strength and freedom. We *are* changing the world. In an unbroken chain from the founding fathers to today, we have been steadily—though not always perfectly—changing the power balance in this country and the world. The old hierarchies are disappearing and the long sweep of history is toward greater individual liberties, not fewer; greater openness and transparency, not less.

Mahatma Ghandi offers gentle words of comfort for those of us who have experienced murder in the name of life, and who now join with all Americans in suffering tragedy at the hands of terrorists:

 When I despair, I remember that all through history the way of truth and love has always won. There have been tyrants and murderers and for a time they seem invincible, but in the end they always fall—think about it, *always.*

But there's a part of me, a part seasoned by decades of trying to protect my staff and my patients, that wants Marti King-Pringle, a retired Planned Parenthood executive, to have the last word in this particular matter:

 We're going to outlast the bastards.

Part IV

Motherhood in freedom

My first baby was due on the twenty-fifth anniversary of *Roe v. Wade*. Throughout my pregnancy, I took every opportunity to tell people my due date and the corresponding anniversary, because I was so proud to have the privilege of giving birth to a girl, the result of a planned and wanted pregnancy, on such an auspicious date.

Our city had a multi-faith service to commemorate the occasion, and as I sat in the chapel listening to the service, I felt my first contraction. I whispered to my colleague who was sitting next to me, and she put her hand on my belly to feel the next contraction. Soon, I had several hands on my belly, and I noticed tears of joy and excitement in the eyes of two of the women touching me, one of whom was a ninety-two-year-old Planned Parenthood volunteer who had endured an illegal abortion in the '40s.

Anti-choice zealots would like to believe that those who support choice have little respect for the miracle of life. Quite the opposite—it is the respect for life that motivates us. Becoming a mother by choice has cemented my belief in the right to choose whether and when to become parents. I remain forever grateful to those who made my choice possible. And I'll spend the rest of my life making sure my daughter and future generations get to keep theirs.

—Tracey, mid-thirties

Chapter Thirteen
Calling ourselves free

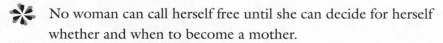 No woman can call herself free until she can decide for herself whether and when to become a mother.

—Margaret Sanger

The liberty of the woman is at stake . . . The mother who carries a child to full term is subject to anxieties, to physical constraints, to pain that only she must bear. That these sacrifices have from the beginning of the human race been endured . . . cannot alone be grounds for the State to insist she make the sacrifice . . . The destiny of the woman must be shaped to a large extent on her own conception of her spiritual imperatives and her place in society.

—*Planned Parenthood of Southeastern Pennsylvania v. Casey*

A job way over my head but straight into my heart

My first day of work in the reproductive health and rights movement was at Permian Basin Planned Parenthood on a hot August day in 1974.

I entered the little two-room, donated office in the American Bank building in downtown Odessa, Texas. Gray steel furniture, no windows. But it was downright luxurious compared to the makeshift classrooms in a Catholic parish hall where I had taught Head Start classes. And a big step up from Patsy Berry's Midland, Texas, garage full of donated condoms and foam where the agency had gotten its start. I was excited and filled with anticipation and eager to get started.

Staff in the "executive office" consisted of me and Mary, a plump, cheery bookkeeper with big hair and a sign on her desk that read "Sexretary." A bright pink and white button on my desk admonished us to "Love Carefully" in those rounded Peter Max letters of the day. Good advice, I thought.

In my office were two boxes of Dalkon Shield IUDs and a note from my predecessor that I should send them back to the manufacturer and get a refund. Other than that, I was pretty much on my own.

The search committee had hired me the night President Nixon resigned. They must have been distracted, or maybe they were just desperate for someone who was a stable resident of West Texas and would stay in the job for more than a year, which had been the tenure of each of the last three executives. I had no health care or administrative experience. I did have a glowing letter of recommendation from my Head Start boss, Mildred Chaffin, written at her suggestion shortly before she died much too young of breast cancer. This would be pure on-the-job training.

I broke out in a rash from stress. But I plunged in.

Today, I get a resumé a week from some bright young person who declares it is her (almost always, it's a her) life's ambition to work for Planned Parenthood. In 1974, it was serendipity not purpose that brought me into the movement.

I was only dimly aware of Margaret Sanger's struggle in the early part of the twentieth century—her nine arrests for providing birth control to bitterly poor women with more children than they could feed. Of Sherri Chessen Finkbine's trip to Sweden for an abortion after taking thalidomide in the 1960s. Of the *Roe v. Wade* decision legalizing abortion, which barely made the front page, competing for attention with Lyndon Johnson's death that same day in 1973. This, even though it was a Texas case argued by a brilliant young Austin attorney, Sarah Weddington.

I did know that the new birth control pill had saved my life in 1962, when I was a twenty-year-old mother of three. I loved my children dearly, but one more just then would have sent me over the edge.

Victims of success

Oblivious to the political context, I thought my job would be running family planning clinics for low-income women in the vast expanses of seventeen West Texas counties. Perhaps I can be excused my political naiveté, as it suffused the movement. It all seemed so simple. Between federal funding for family planning and U.S. Supreme Court decisions legalizing birth control and abortion, it was easy to make a crucial mistake: we thought we had won.

But every victory sows the seeds of the next defeat unless that victory is not just protected but also continuously advanced in new ways by passionate activism equal to that which produced it. At a time when we could have moved swiftly to consolidate our gains, we relied on the courts and avoided the bare-knuckle political fight.

Meanwhile, the same strident opposition that, in the movement's early days, had painted contraception as the devil's work, sure to mean promiscuity and the demise of the family—now shifted its focus to abortion, and we played right into their hands. Many in our movement tried to separate abortion and family planning to minimize controversy in order to protect the family planning service network we had built with such blood, sweat, toil, and tears. "Oh, we don't do abortions here," people would say. "We do family planning."

Separate organizations were formed for the express purpose of advocating for abortion rights in the misguided belief that organizations like Planned Parenthood—with its broader and very mainstream agenda of reproductive health and education services—could stay above the fray. Look how well that worked!

So while we quietly but busily provided the services that allowed individuals to fulfill their dreams of "every child a wanted child," of responsible sexuality, of choice, we didn't notice that the issues were being redefined—and not by us. For on the political battlefield, who-ever defines the issue wins the debate. We couldn't believe there could still be debate about something that made so much sense and helped so many people—and seemed to be supported by everyone, from main-stream clergy to policymakers and, as our polls would later show, the American public.

We were victims of our own success.

And while we talked among ourselves about the best message, we neglected to communicate a broad-based public policy agenda that would mobilize all these individuals to advocate fiercely for all repro-ductive health issues in the political arena. In the void, abortion be-came polarized and sensationalized; sex education and even family planning services became controversial. Once polarized, rational de-bate becomes impossible.

Rights are indivisible—so must advocacy for them be

Both in practice and in law, the same right to privacy underlies access to both birth control and abortion—these rights are indivisible. And once you let fear of controversy deter you from advancing the full mission, you forfeit the moral high ground.

By 1978, I was in Phoenix, Arizona, running Planned Parenthood of Central and Northern Arizona, the affiliate that had been founded in 1937 by Peggy Goldwater with the advice of Margaret Sanger and the full support of Peggy's husband, the future senator. Today's so-called conservatives are sometimes surprised to know that Barry and Peggy were our staunchest supporters. Barry Goldwater believed that a true conservative is pro-choice because he or she wants the government to stay out of something as personal and private as whether and when to have a child.

The attacks increased. Then-PPFA president Faye Wattleton—a charismatic and eloquent speaker—rightly took on the defense of abortion rights full force. But in my view the movement as a whole had become intoxicated with defensive strategies and a sense that the courts would guard our victories. That masked the lack of an equally effective grassroots and policy offensive. And more and more, abortion became the issue while the issues of childbearing choices, access to health care, and reproductive self-determination retreated from the public square. While we worked hard to provide services behind the walls of our clinics, the anti-choice groups were galvanized by their losses. They organized like crazy from the precinct level up. Before the more moderate folks even knew what was happening, the anti-choice insurgents had formed an unholy alliance with the hard-right wing of the Republican Party and had taken control of the party's machinery, though never the hearts and minds of the majority of Republicans. It was guerilla warfare at every policy level.

In Congress, the Hyde amendment outlawed federal funding of abortion for poor women on Medicaid, and the Supreme Court upheld it. If all pro-choice organizations had stood their ground resolutely then, and really mobilized our constituents to fight against this blatant injustice that falls hardest on the backs of the poorest and most vulnerable women, and especially women of color, the course of our history might have been very different.

Talk about moral high ground! What could be more immoral than denying a poor woman who must rely on Medicaid for her health care—and who likely is struggling to get off welfare and become economically self-sufficient—access to abortion if that is her choice? What is fair or just about denying her the autonomy to choose an ethical option that could enable her to take control of her life and take care of her family? This is when it becomes very clear how rights without access are meaningless and why it is necessary to fight against any incursion that would deny access.

Senator Jesse Helms saw to it that no U.S. funds would be spent overseas on abortion and spent much of his long career lambasting the United Nations for its advancement of women's empowerment through reproductive health care.

In the states, minors' access to abortion was the first right to be taken away. Then the states instituted delays for women seeking abortions, and propaganda campaigns that promote childbearing over abortion.

The Reagan "Revolution" of the 1980s, our decade of defensiveness, brought reduced funding for family planning, restrictions on domestic and international family planning services, escalating restrictions on abortion, and a seat at the political table for the extreme, anti-choice right. The courts chipped away at *Roe v. Wade* and opened the door for the states and Congress to do the same. The Reagan-Bush years showed the importance of who is nominating federal judges—and thus the importance of voting your pro-choice convictions every time.

The same legislators, state and federal, who attacked abortion rights also fought family planning and sex education at every turn. They exposed their true anti-woman agenda. If the issue were only about abortion, why wouldn't opponents work with us to reduce unintended pregnancy? But as we have seen, most of these legislators couldn't even be counted on to vote for programs that benefit children or low-income, pregnant women.

In this hostile social and political climate, it was deemed acceptable by the "powers that were" to attack family planning and abortion services and to marginalize and vilify those who provided them. Reproductive health and rights advocates became marginalized in ways both obvious and subtle. The failure of pro-choice leaders and average folks to speak up made them complicit in a growing trend to devalue reproductive rights by painting its advocates as single-issue, a women's issue at that. We were also painted as extremists equivalent to their polar opposites the anti-choice zealots who attack, harass, and worse.

I learn to let no injustice go unchallenged

Here's one small example. Political cartoonist Steve Benson several times characterized me as a murderer. The most egregious of these cartoons depicted Margaret Sanger as Hitler and me as her Gestapo henchman with a Nazi armband motioning people into the gas chamber. This not only offended me as a pro-choice advocate but also as a Jew who lost family members to those gas chambers. It outraged much of the Jewish community. A leading rabbi, Albert Plotkin, whose mother had supported Margaret Sanger's early work, went with me to meet with the editorial board of the newspaper. After hearing our concerns, the editor and Mr. Benson turned to Rabbi Plotkin—literally turning their backs to me—and apologized to him for offending the Jewish community. End of meeting.

It is worth noting that the paper's editor and editorial stance on abortion were soon thereafter changed to more moderate ones. The reasons for that change were many, but I am convinced that even though this meeting brought no apparent gains in the short term, the confrontation had a salutary effect over the long term. And that's why it is so important to let no injustice go unchallenged.

Meanwhile, many community leaders and policymakers, even most clergy, remained silent collaborators when the political and legal attacks devolved into personal harassment and street fighting, and eventually and inevitably into the destruction of clinics . . . and murder.

The escalating violence against clinics where abortions are performed and the doctors who perform them tore at the very fabric of our democracy. The number of abortion providers decreased dramatically. It was mainly the doctors nearing retirement age who remembered what it was like to see a young woman's life snuffed out by illegal and unsafe abortion and who had the will to continue. Medical schools responded to the intimidation by removing abortion training from the women's health curriculum.

Taken together, these policies, laws, court decisions, marginalization, and intimidation placed the greatest burden on those with the least options and power. Although the legal right to privacy remained intact, by the end of the 1990's it was of little value to you if you were young, poor, lived in a rural area, were in or dependent on someone in the military, were in prison, or your hospital was acquired by the sectarian hospital down the street.

The pro-choice Pearl Harbor

The cataclysmic *Webster v. Reproductive Health Services* decision in 1989, opening the doors to substantial state intrusion into childbearing choices, served as a long-needed wake-up call. We had been attacked broadside, and we rose to the occasion, for a while. This was followed in 1992 by *Planned Parenthood v. Casey,* which held that unless a burden was "undue," it could be placed in the path of a woman who has chosen abortion by any legislative body. It allows states to enforce policies that favor childbearing over abortion through propaganda, biased counseling, and mandatory delays. Its underlying assumption is that women have neither the brains nor the hearts and consciences to think about their options and weigh the consequences of their decisions.

So far, few restrictions have been judged "undue."

It was our turn again to organize broadly, to educate and activate—to warn Americans that their personal freedoms had been taken away. I came to understand that we can't fault anti-choice groups for using the democratic process. It is incumbent on us to participate in that process consistently and passionately. Fortunately, there are more of us, so that when we do participate fully, we are sure to prevail.

By 1992, the prevailing political wisdom was that it was better to be pro-choice. The issue was defined as a question of who decides—and it's not the government. We changed the political climate in the states and in Congress—briefly—but we did show that we could do it. Remember the "year of the woman"? We soundly defeated anti-choice ballot initiatives. A pro-choice president was elected, and he eliminated many restrictions on family planning with the stroke of a pen. You could almost hear the collective sigh of pro-choice relief.

In the course of decades of public debate, our values had become bedrock Americana. As people clarified their beliefs about abortion, family planning, and reproductive rights in general, they agreed that women should be able to make their own childbearing decisions. Support for family planning grew to a phenomenal 90 percent. People agreed that prevention is better than punishment. But they didn't translate that personal belief into political action unless there was a direct "Pearl Harbor" assault that they could see and feel. As one woman caller who decried the complacency said to me when I was on a radio show to discuss the fortieth anniversary of the birth control pill, "My daughter thinks the pill is like the air, all around her, always there when she wants it."

A movement has to move

Our very effective but defensive "who decides?" message was a narrow libertarian appeal that got people riled up when they perceived an imminent threat. But in the end, it reduced the issue to abortion once again and ducked the profound moral questions of whose life and whose conscience counts, as well as the policy questions of fairness, equity, and access. It forfeited the language of values. It allowed the onslaught against a woman's right to have a life, and a child's right to have a decent future, to go on, inadequately challenged.

Without an affirmative agenda—an agenda sufficient to inspire an activist movement absent a perceived, immediate threat—a defensive message alone could not keep pro-choice constituents mobilized. We —all of us—need something to aspire to as well as something to fear. In the main, after 1992, people sat back down, snug in the knowledge that the veto pen would protect them.

And then came 1994, the Gingrich revolution, the "Contract with (or 'on') America," and renewed attacks of all kinds. What might have been years of triumph became instead the lowest ebb of the movement in at least the last decade.

My years in the maelstrom of state politics had taught me that the only way to get out of this downward spiral is to change the field of play to one where we can set the agenda and fight on those vast playing fields where we are so strong. This is not to say there were no proactive policy initiatives during this era. The Freedom of Choice Act, for example, aimed to codify reproductive rights. It never received a full vote, felled both by opposition and by disagreements about language among pro-choice leaders. And the Freedom of Access to Clinics Entrances Act was passed and signed into law, bringing greater protections for reproductive health providers. But there were many more initiatives attacking abortion and family planning at the federal, state, and local levels. We just simply had to change our mindset from the thermometer to the thermostat.

It is much more energizing to have a positive policy agenda. And there is every reason to advance such an agenda. So much remains to be done in a country where insurance covers Viagra more often than the Pill; where medically accurate, comprehensive sexuality education essentially doesn't exist; where women who are raped are denied emergency contraception in hospital emergency rooms.

In 1996, eighty years after Margaret Sanger opened her first birth control clinic, I accepted my greatest challenge, the presidency of Planned Parenthood Federation of America, at a time when the organization's finances and morale were dismal. Talk about going from the frying pan into the fire.

After twenty-two years of leading affiliates, I felt I had made my contribution. I had planned to retire for a couple of years to write and travel with my husband. But when I was recruited for this position, and encouraged by so many people around the country, I knew that it was a perfect fit in spite of the huge challenges and the personal sacrifices my family and I would have to make. Alex, especially, deserves a medal for uprooting himself from the new house he loved, retiring from the business he had built, and building a new life in New York (where he had vowed he'd never live again).

During the latter stages of the search process, Alex and I had what would be our last real vacation for some time, hiking the Milford Track in New Zealand. It is an incredibly beautiful thirty-three-mile hike, but once you get started, there can be no turning back. What I remember most is having to gather the courage, in spite of my terror, to cross the Track's twenty-two rudimentary rope and wire bridges suspended over vast gorges and raging rivers. That was excellent preparation for what was awaiting me!

My first message to our stakeholders was that a good defense is necessary but clearly not sufficient. We must be thermostats, not thermometers; we must create the social climate rather than merely respond to it. Reproductive health services should be everywhere, available and accessible to all who need them in whatever form they need them. The Internet is a good metaphor for how all of our services need to be everywhere and available to all. We must organize and mobilize this nationwide movement, its grassroots and influential activist base, around a constantly invigorated policy agenda that challenges the injustices and enables us to create exciting new programs and services that people want and need.

A movement has to move. Power and energy come from moving into new places, not staying where you are or going backwards. The birth control movement was born from the courageous leadership of Margaret Sanger. When she opened the first family planning clinic, she took a dramatic political action that called attention to the heart-rending stories of women, and in so doing, began the process of changing the laws. Today, only equally dramatic political action can ensure that the women and men of tomorrow will continue to have access to the reproductive health and education services we've struggled to build and provide.

We should take heart from our success in reducing unintended pregnancy and teen pregnancy substantially, even though both remain far too high. We should take courage from the national groundswell toward contraceptive equity in health insurance, a movement we created to rectify a modern injustice. Those are just two examples of successes that should inspire many more future initiatives.

This movement is ready to soar

When I think about the history of our movement, I am struck not by the obstacles in our path today but by how far we have come since our beginnings. Our resolve has remained constant, but the stakes are so much higher, so our responsibilities have escalated. A movement or an organization that fails to evolve will wither and die. That's why we are looking ahead and defining the future. And that's why, having now built practical systems and the forward-looking agenda to support a growing group of activists, this movement is ready to soar. And it is about time. Let us be clear about what's at stake. My right to choose abortion is equal to your right to use birth control is equal to your neighbor's right to have a child, and none of it should be decided by anyone except ourselves.

Roe v. Wade is at great risk. And the same legal theory that underlies *Roe* is also the basis for the Supreme Court's landmark *Griswold v. Connecticut* decision in 1965. That decision made birth control legal for married people, nullifying the Comstock laws under which Margaret Sanger was prosecuted for distributing information about contraception and articulating a right to privacy in childbearing decisions. In between came *Eisenstadt v. Baird,* establishing that "If the right of privacy means anything, it is the right of individuals, married or single, to be free from unwarranted government intrusion into matters so fundamentally affecting a person as the decision whether to bear or beget a child."

So it is not a stretch to say that if abortion rights go, birth control rights are equally at risk. Both are built upon the same legal principle of reproductive privacy. Both could revert to being at the whim of legislative bodies. In fact, many states have never repealed their old, pre-*Roe* and *Griswold* laws.

But this time it would be much worse than in the days before 1973, when the states weighed in with their restrictions but the federal government largely kept out of it. Congress is in the act now. And the political machinery of the anti-choice groups is well oiled and ready to take advantage of any opportunity.

Further, we face adversaries who are smart, well funded, and zealously determined to prevail. They have a friend in the White House who has put his friends in charge of the Department of Justice and the Department of Health and Human Services' octopus-like tentacles reaching into a myriad of health and education offices that touch every American's life.

Since his first day in office, President George W. Bush and his appointees, alongside the anti-choice members of Congress, and aided and abetted by the now inside groups of the anti-choice far right, have been on a mission to undermine decades of progress and to roll back the reproductive rights of women here in the U.S. and around the globe. I would call their alliance the "axis of anti-choice evil." But an axis only connects its elements. The overt and covert actions of the anti-choice policymakers today are weaving a pernicious web of anti-choice evil. The individual strands might look fragile, but woven together, will soon ensnare and strangle the basic human right to freedom of childbearing choice if we do not rip them away swiftly and surely. I have described some of these grave threats in previous chapters, but I'll put them together here:

> Censoring free speech—On his first full day in office, Bush imposed the undemocratic global gag rule on international family planning programs, risking the lives of millions of women and children living in misery and destitution. Domestic gag rules are already at hand in some states and spreading rapidly to others.

> Reducing access to family planning and real sex education services—Bush defied Congress and stripped the United Nations Population Fund of U.S dollars that had been appropriated. (His 2002 budget had even eliminated contraceptive

coverage for federal employees, but Congress soundly rebuffed this mean-spirited policy.) Funding for dangerous and irresponsible abstinence-only sex education programs has escalated, and if the president's 2003 budget passes intact, will total almost $150 million a year. Meanwhile, dollars allocated to Title X family planning services for low-income women reach less than half those who would be eligible.

➤ Redefining the status of the fetus in law—New federal regulations play the cruel game of declaring fetuses children from the moment of conception and making them—not pregnant women—eligible for prenatal care under the State Child Health Insurance Program. This may sound like a ho-hum, harmless thing to do, but it is flat out an attempt to elevate the fetus to primacy in law, over the status of the woman. Similarly, proposed state and federal laws attempt to give the fetus separate personhood status in criminal law when harm to a pregnant woman creates harm to her fetus, and even to apply the laws of adoption to frozen embryos.

➤ Building the platform to overturn *Roe*—John Ashcroft's Department of Justice took the unusual step of weighing in on the side of the state in a case pending before the Sixth Circuit Court of Appeals. The case seeks to overturn an Ohio district court's decision that struck down the state's abortion ban—or so-called "partial birth abortion" law—as unconstitutional. This after Ashcroft swore under oath that *Roe* is settled law and he would enforce it.

➤ Shaping the courts so they will be prepared to overturn *Roe* and create new legal precedents to end the fundamental right to reproductive self-determination—Packing the federal courts at all levels with anti-choice judges is the final thread in the pernicious web that can end reproductive rights—signed, sealed, and strangled. The Bush administration will make the critical appointments to the U. S. Supreme Court, which stands one tenuous vote away from overturning *Roe*. Even if reproductive rights remain theoretically intact, they won't mean a thing without full and unfettered access to the information and services that make them real.

Advancing a spectacular offensive: An agenda for the twenty-first century

The twentieth century brought a sea change in women's lives, thanks to the many leaders and ordinary citizens who changed laws, devised better technology, and created a service network. Now, the great challenge of the twenty-first century is to elevate women's reproductive self-determination to the same level as other cherished, fundamental human and civil rights, and to make access to reproductive health and education services universal in the U.S. and globally.

To do so, we must advance an affirmative agenda—a spectacular offensive—to achieve our victories, to fight on the battlefields where we define the terms of engagement, to give pro-choice constituents something to aspire to as well as something to fear, to keep the movement moving forward, in order to fulfill our commitment to make *every* child a wanted child and every woman free to define her own life.

We must deliver our visionary message about what the world will look like when our positive agenda is fulfilled, providing nothing less than hope for humanity: the freedom to dream, to make choices, and to live in peace with our planet. Every pro-choice person must consider it his or her responsibility to speak up and out to deliver that message, for a movement is only as strong as the will of its individual members.

We must use the best technology to organize the American majority who support this cause and to engage them in the democratic process. We must especially educate and mentor and connect to this movement each new generation who risks taking reproductive freedom for granted and who has the most at stake if it is lost.

We must leverage our commitment to diversity to make common cause with other groups who have also been marginalized, so that we may capitalize on our collective power and influence for the common good. For we understand that embracing the rich diversity of humanity is a necessary condition to achieving the social justice and equality we seek for women.

We must make sex a good word. We must engender healthier, more realistic attitudes about sexuality in our culture in order to reduce our dismal rates of unintended pregnancy, teen pregnancy, and sexually transmitted infections.

We must control the means of producing and distributing our messages, our materials, and the outstanding reproductive health and sexuality education programming that is so often censored today. Simultaneously we must challenge the mass media to be more responsible about the images it portrays and to break down its barriers to contraceptive advertising.

Abortion must be put back where it belongs in the core of women's health care.

The fundamental right to make our own childbearing choices must be guaranteed by the U.S. Constitution and state and federal laws.

New technologies like mifepristone and emergency contraception must be supported and brought into the health care system without barriers. There is the promise of new fertility treatments to help couples trying to conceive, and a vast need to increase research funding for new contraceptives. Reproductive options are multiplying and becoming more complex, so we must lead the public debate through the ethical ramifications as well as the medical ones in a principled, not a polarized, way.

Ominous and powerful forces are arrayed against the laws and services that enabled Crissy—the young woman whose story introduces this book—to make her dreams come true. The biggest challenge by far is that the majority of Americans cannot believe this fact—yet. So our movement's political entities must aggressively connect the dots between public opinion and citizen behavior to deliver the pro-choice votes that support pro-choice politicians and defeat anti-choice politicians.

We must create a social climate in which policymakers of all parties find it in their best interest to support family planning, medically accurate and comprehensive sex education, and abortion rights without weaseling or waffling.

We must build the most formidable activist base anywhere. Too many pro-choice voters still simply cannot imagine that choice could disappear—so they think they need not make it a deciding factor in how they vote. "It's not an issue," I hear over and over, "We've already won." Then there is sheer denial: "They couldn't really take us backward." And an entire generation has grown up having no experience of life without choice—just as we'd hoped they would.

Well, start imagining. It *is* an issue. Choice *can* disappear. You'd better believe it can. And there's so much more we need to do to guarantee access to the full range of reproductive and sexual health care to all.

For as long as there are unintended pregnancies, as long as there is HIV/AIDS, as long as pregnancy sentences teens to poverty and dependency, reproductive choice is an issue. Until no person can hope to be appointed to the U.S. Supreme Court or any court unless he or she expresses firm support of the human and civil right to reproductive self-determination, it is an issue. Until every human on the face of the earth has the information needed to make responsible choices about sex, pregnancy, and childbearing, until no woman dies from unsafe abortion or too many pregnancies in this world, until all pregnancies are the result of love and planning, until every child is wanted and loved, until we can all call ourselves free, it is an issue.

And once we've achieved all that—another generation will be born, and we'll start all over to ensure they have the same future. The minute we sit back and say we've won, the momentum and the moment whistle by us.

I have been there and I have done that. And I am determined it will not happen again. I am joined in this conviction by my extraordinary, courageous, strong, persistent, and increasingly energized colleagues in this movement. We have been through the crucible. We have honed our skills and our convictions. We are fierce and fearless. We are prepared to change the social climate once and for all to one that is actively supportive of reproductive rights and health care.

Defining moments

People sometimes ask if there was a defining moment when I knew this would be my passion, my life's work.

From the day I walked into that tiny office, I sensed that my entire value system, articulated or not, conscious or not, was in sync with Planned Parenthood's. Preventing unintended pregnancy was a natural outgrowth of my previous Head Start work to improve the lot of poor children and their families. I placed a high priority on education, and fought for civil rights and social justice, for women in particular. As I pursued my own education, I had become concerned about over-population and environmental degradation. My religion encouraged me to try to improve the world around me. I knew that a woman can't control any aspect of her life if she can't control her fertility—and she shouldn't have to forgo her sexuality to do so.

I knew the hardships and deficits of being a teen parent, a young mother who could not have another child and still care adequately for those I already had. I still get a lump of burning anger in my throat when I see anyone judging someone else's decision about something so personal as childbearing. Planned Parenthood just made so much sense in all respects—from the most intensely individual to the global.

It was integrity of belief and experience and values personified in a job. I was lucky and I knew it, in spite of the rash.

Important events in the struggle for reproductive self-determination

➤ 1848—The first women's rights convention is held in Seneca Falls, New York. The world's population is about to reach one billion.

➤ 1873—Anthony Comstock, who saw vice everywhere he looked, succeeds in criminalizing the dissemination of birth control information and materials, labeling them as obscene.

➤ 1916—Margaret Sanger opens a birth control clinic in Brooklyn, the first in the U.S. She is indicted and arrested for violation of the Comstock law, but the birth control movement is launched.

➤ 1920—Women in the U.S. win the right to vote.

➤ 1937—The American Medical Association acknowledges that birth control should be taught in medical schools.

➤ 1942—The Planned Parenthood Federation of America is formed.

➤ 1952—The Planned Parenthood Federation of America is co-founder of the International Planned Parenthood Federation.

➤ 1953—Katherine Dexter McCormick makes the first of many contributions, eventually totally $2 million, to fund development of an oral contraceptive.

➤ 1960—Finally. Hormonal contraception (quickly and everlastingly dubbed "The Pill")—saves the sanity and health of American women.

➤ 1963—She had been administered thalidomide, which causes birth defects, but Sherri (Chessen) Finkbine is refused an abortion in Phoenix, Arizona. Her gravely deformed fetus is aborted in Sweden, and her story convinces many of the need to legalize abortion in the U.S.

➤ 1964—The Civil Rights Act prohibits employers from discriminating on the basis of race, creed, national origin, or sex.

➤ 1965—In *Griswold v. Connecticut,* the U.S. Supreme Court rules that laws that prohibit the use of birth control are unconstitutional as a violation of the right of privacy.

➤ 1970—Congress enacts Title X of the Public Health Services Act, which provides family planning for low-income women and teens. Hawaii and New York become first states to repeal criminal abortion laws.

➤ 1972—*Eisenstadt v. Baird* makes it legal for unmarried people to obtain birth control. The U.S. Senate sends the Equal Rights Amendment to the states for ratification.

➤ 1973—Ruling in *Roe v. Wade*, the U.S. Supreme Court extends the right to privacy to include abortion, declaring that state laws restricting that right are unconstitutional. The National Right to Life committee is first convened in reaction.

➤ 1976—Congress passes the first Hyde Amendment, prohibiting the use of Medicaid funds for abortion while continuing to fund childbirth.

➤ 1982—On the deadline for its ratification, the Equal Rights Amendment fails, three states short of ratification.

➤ 1985—President Ronald Reagan issues executive order placing a gag rule on international family planning funds by instituting the so-called "Mexico City Policy" that denies funding to nongovernmental organizations that provide, counsel, or refer for abortion with non-U.S. government funds.

➤ 1987—Ronald Reagan tries to "gag" domestic family planning providers by tying their family planning funding to silence on the subject of abortion.

➤ 1989—*Webster v. Reproductive Health Services* allows substantial state interference with a woman's ability to exercise her right to an abortion, and sets the scene for a possible reversal of *Roe v. Wade*.

➤ 1992—In *Planned Parenthood of Southeastern Pennsylvania v. Casey*, the U.S. Supreme Court further weakens the Constitutional protections of *Roe*, allowing states to impose such restrictions as mandatory delays and anti-choice propaganda, claiming they do not impose an "undue burden." In "The Year of the Woman," more women than ever run for and are elected to office, and a pro-choice president is elected.

➤ 1993—Bill Clinton is inaugurated president of the U.S. and eliminates gag rules and the ban on importation of mifepristone for research purposes. Dr. David Gunn is assassinated by anti-choice terrorists.

➤ 1994—More than 160 nations agree upon a Programme of Action at the United Nations International Conference on Population and Development in Cairo. The Programme highlights women's empowerment and reproductive health as key to global well-being and population stabilization.

➤ 1997—The Equity in Prescription Insurance and Contraceptive Coverage Act is first introduced in Congress.

➤ 1999—World population reaches six billion.

➤ 2000—Mifepristone, a medical alternative to surgical abortion, is approved for use in the U.S. The U.S. Supreme Court rules five to four in *Stenberg v. Carhart* a woman's health must be considered in restricting access to abortion. George W. Bush, promising anti-choice policies, is elected president in a demonstration of the power of one U.S. Supreme Court justice's vote and thus the importance of who has the power of appointment.

➤ 2001—Bush wasn't kidding. His first official act is to impose the global gag rule. *Erickson v. Bartell* establishes contraceptive coverage as gender equity.

➤ 2002—Pro-choice state and federal initiatives advance contraceptive coverage, emergency contraception access, and real sex education, supported by the vast majority of voters.

Vision for 2025—The pro-choice movement masses its strength and engages its activists in the democratic process. There are social climates, laws, and policies that support reproductive choice, and everyone has full access to reproductive and sexual health care and education.

Chapter Fourteen

"We aren't the future, we're the present"

I once made the mistake of calling young people "the future" of the family planning movement. The teens in the audience answered in no uncertain terms: "We aren't the future, we're the present." But what does the present mean to them? What meaning will they give to reproductive rights?

From generation to generation

One thing we know: sex isn't a disease that gets cured once and for all. Each new generation has its own timetable for maturity and its own definition of relationships. Each generation defines family planning and reproductive self-determination in its own ways and asks different things of this movement.

This is how meaning has evolved over the last three generations. A couple of years ago I visited Lincoln, Nebraska, to speak at an event. I met a ninety-five-year-old woman who came because she wanted to tell me personally that she got a diaphragm from Margaret Sanger's clinic when she was a young wife. It was during the Depression, and she simply couldn't afford more children. For her, reproductive rights meant the relief of knowing that she would be able to take care of the children she already had, and she could stop having further pregnancies. She was brought to the lunch by her sixtyish daughter and son-in-law. They told me that family planning had allowed them to finish graduate school. It enabled them to delay having children, and it meant the freedom to enjoy their sexual love without pregnancy. They had to go to a neighboring state to get birth control because it was still illegal where they went to college, but they knew about it and they were determined to have this measure of control over their lives. This couple brought with them their son and daughter-in-law, thirty-somethings who had recently adopted a baby. The young couple wanted to talk to me about how family planning, to them, means assuring the full range of options and an opportunity to nurture a child.

The underlying values remain the same: the freedom to plan a family. But everything else changes over time, as the story of the three generations richly illustrates. The women who today are the age of those who came to Margaret Sanger to quit having children, now visit family planning clinics before they have their very first pregnancy and can plan thoughtfully and joyously for that day.

What does the next generation ask from family planning providers and the reproductive rights movement—the young women and men just now thinking about forming their families? And what can the rest of us learn from them? When the global "youth quake" generation rocks the planet, what will everyone's quality of life be? And what is this Britney Spears idealization of virginity while writhing with sexual invitation, anyway?

Hands on, concrete, grass-roots

Today's young people are active and involved—but in different ways than their elders. They don't want to pay membership fees and sit on boards—they want to educate themselves about the issues and join a grassroots network. They don't want to come to meetings and manage volunteers—they want to help in concrete, personal, hands-on ways.

I was especially taken by the compassionate words of this budding physician:

 After several years of counseling patients who were considering having an abortion, I learned that there truly is a story behind every choice. Whether it's the woman's first pregnancy or fifth abortion; whether she's fourteen or forty-two; whether the conception is the result of rape or marital bliss; if she doesn't want to have this particular baby right now, how could I want her to? How could that be what's best for her health or what's right for the potential child inside of her? A pregnancy can be the most exciting thing a woman ever experiences or the most terrifying, and each case is unique, medically and emotionally.

I hope to become an obstetrician and to have the privilege of offering women my support and assistance, whatever their choice regarding pregnancy—avoiding it, achieving it, nurturing it, or discontinuing it. I feel extremely grateful to live in a time when that vision, that every child be a wanted child, is practically possible. What the next generation needs is health care providers who are able and willing to provide abortions as part of a full range of women's health care services, rather than relegating that work to a few isolated "abortionists." We need providers who can say to their patients, "I will help you, whatever your choice."

—Elizabeth, age twenty-five

I share their enthusiasm for the grassroots approach to political action. I first experienced its power as a teenager, thanks to a boy named Ralph, and I often tell young people this story to illustrate the power they have in their hands. In my teenage years in Stamford, Texas, we all hung out at Son's City Pig. We went through phases, as teenagers do, of eating strange things like mustard with our French fries. The crotchety man who owned the place was named "Son" and we called him "Mr.

Son." Mr. Son was annoyed with us for asking for mustard, and probably he was annoyed with us in general for being rambunctious teenagers. He started charging us two cents for mustard.

This, we thought, was a moral outrage. Ralph gathered a dozen or so of us together out on the parking lot and suggested that we go then and there to talk with Mr. Jackson, who owned a drive-in across town called the Superdog. We all piled into two cars and drove to the Superdog. Ralph went in and asked Mr. Jackson to come out to the parking lot and talk with us because there was no place to sit down inside. We proceeded to tell Mr. Jackson that if he would build a room where we could sit down, install a jukebox, and give us free mustard, we and all our friends would bring our business to him. Smart man, he quickly agreed. The Superdog became our hangout. We were happy and Mr. Jackson prospered. Son's City Pig went out of business a couple of years later.

The world has changed a lot since Ralph and Mr. Son implemented their very different business plans. Today, young people do their grassroots organizing over the Internet—a powerful tool that gives them enormous opportunity—and responsibility. They can do much more than achieve a place to dance and get free mustard. They truly have the ability to change the world.

It will take the kind of determination that Jenny describes in her story:

 At fourteen, a girl has no idea what to do or where to turn if she gets pregnant. I was this fourteen-year-old girl who ended up pregnant and found I was completely unknowing of what to do and where to go for help. But, I have an amazing family who helped me through the entire situation and even the years after it when I dealt with the issue of abortion on an intensely emotional and personal level.

So, as the years passed and I grew up, I gained my own views and developed my own opinions of abortion and a woman's right to her reproductive freedom. I can't help but think, and even shudder at the thought, that at one time in history there were other 14-year-old girls who got pregnant and weren't so lucky as I. All these girls had available to them were the "Back Alley Abortions." Some lived through it, others died. Just think, without continued action to keep "A Woman's Right to Choose" alive, we may find that someday, in the not so distant future, it just may be one of our fourteen-year-old daughters' who has no reproductive rights and has to go into the "Back Alley." Funny, but I thought times were supposed to move ahead for the better. I, as a woman who was blessed to have my freedom of choice, intend to continue doing all I can to keep *all* women safe . . . and their daughters . . . and granddaughters, too.

Mentor us

We have perhaps taken for granted that young people, who have the most at stake, would automatically gravitate to this movement. But there is so much more we must do to fuel their passion for the reproductive rights and health agenda. The generation born after *Roe* does not know about coat hangers as an instrument for self-induced abortion, nor do we want them to. But they are asking to hear the story from us, and they must find themselves in the story.

Amanika Kumar, who became a pro-choice volunteer while still a teenager and is now a college student, says this:

 All young adults look for this kind of guidance from their elders to teach them how to go where they want to go. And if they do not find it, they will take the easier path of ignorance and apathy. Whether it is by talking to adults or following their example, young adults long for and seek the mentorship of those adults who they trust and admire. Mentorship is an integral part of creating our future. As we all know, the time has come to start thinking of the future of reproductive rights and pass the torch to the next generation of activists. But before we can do that, we must cultivate the support of my generation.

Byllye Avery, founder of the National Black Women's Health Project and a longtime women's rights activist, suggests that "women who bleed" should take up this movement. It seems to me that in a sense, all women will bleed, as will the increasing number of men who care about women's reproductive rights, until together we have infused our culture with the policies and services that guarantee reproductive rights once and for all. As Beth, who was eighteen in 1969 when she became pregnant unintentionally and still remembers how frightened she was when she bled profusely after an illegal abortion, put it:

 It's a profound thing. As a woman you have the power to give life and the power to take it away. And you can't pretend that you don 't. I've always said that until sexism is gone, you can't deny women the right to an abortion. If there hadn't been sexism, I would have been able to get good information, birth control would have been accessible, and I wouldn't have felt coerced. I don't mean that the guy I was with coerced me, but the culture coerced me. I would never have felt like it was all up to me and that I alone was responsible to do something. I could have said that I didn't want to get pregnant so we are going to do this, to make sure that I don't become pregnant. I'm an optimist so I think someday sexism will be gone, but I don't think any time soon.

I know what Byllye means, though, and she's right that it is time for younger women and men to take up this cause for their own sakes. There will always be a new generation coming on that needs the information, the sexuality education, the medical services, the birth control methods, the help and support to make those important life decisions.

I guess it's human nature to think you are indispensable, to try to continue to own something to which you've devoted so much of yourself. But movements only live if they continue to move. And the greatest honor bestowed upon me recently has been having two extraordinary, bright, and committed young women (one seventeen and one in her early twenties) each declare publicly that she wants my job. Things won't stay the same, not by a long shot. Nor should they.

How annoyed I was when I heard the young feminist writer, Jennifer Baumgardner, co-author of *Manifesta,* claim that the problem with pro-choice women my age is that we fight only the defensive battles when we should be advancing legislation like contraceptive coverage (after all, I've personally spent years pushing that rock of proactivism up the hill of complacency and have made contraceptive coverage practically my signature initiative). Then I remembered: Each generation has to say things themselves in their own way and each generation has to push against the last. It is actually a compliment that Jennifer uses that example and I am happy as a clam that she feels she owns it. That ownership guarantees the movement will grow and thrive.

One thing seems clear and gives me great optimism—they, more than my generation or the one after me or the one before me, really get it. The young people who are getting involved with this movement understand the full implications of fertility control. The implications for men as well as women. For the earth that we share. For self-esteem, for life skills, for the definition of family. For the ability of women and all people to be all that they can be.

 Today, at age thirty—and still childless by choice—I look back on that twenty-three-year old woman [when she became pregnant unintentionally and had an abortion]. Today I do not take the right to choose for granted. Today I respect myself and would not dream of taking part in a relationship that does not include mutual respect. Today I know that my reproductive rights are not something to play around with, because the right to procreate or not procreate is not a game. The next generation needs to know that people have not marched in the streets and passed laws to secure the reproductive freedoms of all women just so that many of us can throw caution to the wind where our bodies or liberties are concerned. This goes out to all the guys too, particularly those who complain about using condoms. You guys have a choice to make as well. You can do the smart thing or deal with much more difficult choices later. The next generation needs a stronger sense of inner value instilled. Value of their bodies and minds and of the future generations they bring into this world. Abortion is a reproductive choice, and it always should be, but it is nothing to be taken lightly any more than the decision to have a child.

—Erin, age thirty

Those of us who fought and still fight to banish forever the specter of back-alley abortions from our land can be proud. We have freed today's young people to see the big picture, to view reproductive health care holistically, to be concerned about women and families all over the world. They understand that the "youth quake" generation coming of age in developing countries not only faces an uncertain future due to lack of family planning but also a fragile planet. They express concerns not just for women's rights but for the fulfillment of the physical and emotional needs of men and women, children and elders, people of all sexual orientations:

 We need to start looking at this issue as one that involves the self worth of every one. From girls and women, to boys and men. When one speaks of reproductive rights in the future, it will mean that our political system and our communities must support every program and effort to help all persons make informed choices about their lives. These choices start when children are young. The choices range from being able to get a good education, adequate nutrition, affordable housing, access to a wide range of healthcare, job training, choosing a career path, and being able to amass financial security. It means supporting effective after school programs, libraries, parks, and helping everyone to develop their spiritual self.

It will be necessary to support measures that make contraception available to every person having sex. Most importantly, we must support parents to speak openly with their children about sex in a caring and understanding way. Abortion must be seen as a safe procedure that should stay legal. Reproductive rights is a holistic issue, much more than being either pro choice or anti abortion. If we do that, then we are missing the other 9/10ths of the struggle, which is to create individuals with self worth and dignity. Without those two things, the cycle of unplanned pregnancy will forever mar the futures of countless girls, women, boys and men.

—Vanessa, age twenty-two

Margaret Sanger was riveted by the voice of Sadie Sachs, who had been told by her doctor that she should tell her husband, Jake, to sleep on the roof, if she didn't want more children. While I heard the voices of women wanting to plan their families, space their children, and never return to the days of illegal abortion, the young people of today can hear all of the voices of all of the people who are seeking better lives, and they tend to zero in on helping them one at a time. They are engaged on campuses, and off, in getting access to emergency contraception, changing medical school training, ending violence against women, demanding that their insurance plans cover contraception, and much more.

Hope for humanity incarnate

In the voices of these young people, I hear hope for the future:

Limitations can no longer be permitted. If a young woman wishes to purchase birth control, we have to make it available for her to purchase/obtain with little or no hassle. If a young lesbian woman wants to get a pap smear and feels unable to do so because of the fear of being 'outed,' there is obviously a problem. Education is ultimately the key component. Without educating young women and men about their options, choices available to them, and services they can obtain, we really are not making progress.

—Jolene, age twenty-one

 Through education we can give the future generations the tools to make decisions that are right for them. One of the worst crimes that we can commit against the future of reproductive choice is to throw our arms up and proclaim, "You know, it just doesn't have anything to do with me!" Generate your own light to make up for the blown fuses of those who don't understand that a choice is a basic human need. You've got your whole life ahead of you, but remember, that's not a very long time in the scale of things. It's up to everyone that comes after us to keep it all going.

—Hollie, age twenty-seven

As our younger sisters, and brothers, too, take up the mantle, we must ensure they understand that the struggle to secure the rights that so many now take for granted was fueled by the blood of women who, in quiet acts of individual courage, risked their lives and health for their families and their futures.

Here's how Amanika puts it:

 You, the past and current leaders of the struggle for reproductive rights, need to teach us. We don't know what it was like thirty, thirty-five, forty years ago. You need to tell us, because if you don't tell us the past, we are doomed to repeat it. You are our best connection to our past fight for reproductive rights. Teach us. I am asking you to join with me and the others committed to our struggle and mentorship to take simple steps to educate my generation. It will be a slow process with baby steps, but we are the beginning grass roots of an important fight. If we don't join now to ensure a future of human and reproductive rights, we are destined for a future without them.

And as we tell our stories, we can be sure they will make a difference, as this young woman's words affirm:

 I came of age long after *Roe v. Wade* made abortion legal, and have gone through most of my twenties taking my right to get birth control and reproductive services for granted. I recently saw a video called "Before Abortion was Legal"—it was this compilation of women telling stories about the horrible things they did to their bodies or helped their friends do before 1973. The quiet way they told their stories just underlined the horror and wretchedness of the desperate lengths that they had gone to. I reached a point where I had to turn off the tape because it affected me so emotionally. I decided right then that no woman I love—my mother, my sister, my best friend—should ever have to go through that to obtain basic health care. I've since become more knowledgeable about all the threats to our rights: pending court cases that may overturn Roe, the manufacture of the "partial-birth abortion" issue by extremist groups, the lack of contraceptive coverage in my insurance policy. etc. I will always trace my activism back to that moment.

—Robin, age twenty-four

We light many torches to make the future bright

As we not only pass the torch, but light enough new ones to illuminate the path for all men and women and children, here and around the world—as we recognize that the stories and the choices of the next generation may be very different from ours but no less valid—as we challenge and as we encourage them to know and share their own stories, we must never forget. For Amanika and all the other young people who have asked to understand the history and meaning of this movement, I offer this story of three generations as instruction and inspiration:

 I used contraception successfully for thirty-five years. I was lucky in that it never failed me. I had one planned pregnancy that ended in a miscarriage. My husband and I then spent many years in a thoughtful process which led to a decision to remain childless by choice. Although it is about empowerment and self-determination, mine is a boring story in the telling. But the stories of the shoulders I stood on so I could be so smart are the ones worth telling. I always knew my mother had had an illegal abortion. She never told me, I just knew. I don't even remember how I knew there was such a thing as abortion—I just knew that too. The social mores of her time inhibited my mother from telling me about birth control, but she did say—"if you ever get in trouble, promise me you'll come to me and not a stranger." It was the early 1960s and abortion was illegal.

Decades later, I finally had the guts to ask my mother about her abortion. When my apolitical mother asked to join my husband Peter and me on the March in Washington the April before the Webster decision, I asked her if it was to finally reconcile her feelings around her illegal abortion. She looked at me as if I had two heads. No, she said, it is to ensure that my granddaughters never have to endure what I did. Well, I felt stupid.

My not asking her the details of her abortion all those years was my problem, not hers. So one night, I finally asked her to tell me her story, over a bottle of wine and dinner in her apartment.

It was the end of the depression. Jobs were scarce and housing unaffordable. My mother's job in a book bindery would be at risk if she married. When she and my father discovered she was pregnant, they decided abortion was the right course of action for them at that time. My mother's brother was a cop and he knew where to go. My mother and father went to an apartment where a "nice" woman calling herself a nurse inserted a stiff rod of some kind into my mother 's cervix after she climbed onto something she remembers as resembling an ironing board. The "rod" may have been glass or stiff rubber tubing. The "nurse" told her that she would cramp and bleed within forty-eight hours. My mother left with the rod in her, went to work the next day and miscarried by herself in the ladies room. She was athletic and strong and in very good health, and she was sure that helped her get through it without complications. She cleaned herself up and went back to work. She doesn't remember much else. She still maintains that she was "lucky" when she thinks about what other women went through. Then my mother took me completely by surprise and told me something I did not know. My grandmother Anna, an immigrant from Eastern Europe and a devout Roman Catholic with seven children, had almost died from the complications of an illegal septic abortion. Her daughter Helen, my mother, stood at her bedside in the hospital at the age of twelve as the authorities tried to question her very ill mother. My grandmother was in a coma for a long time and in the hospital for months; she was given the last rites. There was no health insurance then, and the mounting bills led to my grandparents losing their home.

In the years since that dinner, my mother has given me permission to use her story in speeches and writings. On the occasion of the Twenty-fifth Anniversary of the *Roe* decision, she allowed her story and my grandmother's to be featured in an op ed that appeared in the *Philadelphia Inquirer.* She lives in a very conservative area, in a seniors' apartment building. The author said it was important to use my mother's full name to "make her real." I warned my mother that she might get some harassment. At eighty-four, Helen Sartori said it was the most important thing she had ever done, and easily gave her permission.

When Helen Sartori went public with her story, she told her daughter, Joan Coombs—a woman who has devoted her life to this movement—that she did it in her honor. And so it goes, from generation to generation, and always will.

Present tense—resources for young people

The Internet is today's Son's City Pig, where young people hang out and grassroots organizing takes place. It's easier, faster and less fattening. Planned Parenthood resources for information about reproductive health care and advocacy for reproductive rights include:

➤ **www.plannedparenthood.org,** which contains the latest information on public policy and sexual health, plus fact sheets, guides to sexuality education, and links to other sites. **www.plannedparenthood.org/action** takes you directly to advocacy information and lets you sign up for breaking news and action charts.

➤ *Vox* is organized especially for young people who want to get involved in protecting reproductive rights. There are local chapters on college campuses and affiliated with Planned Parenthood in your area. Visit **www.plannedparenthood.org/vox.**

➤ Questions about sex, human development, relationships and more can be answered at **www.teenwire.com**. The safe place in cyberspace for teens.

➤ Go directly to **www.saveroe.com** for the latest action items on reproductive rights in general or to **www.covermypills.com** to learn how you can further contraceptive equity.

➤ Reproductive health services are available at Planned Parenthood throughout the U.S. Find the clinic nearest you by calling 1-800-230-PLAN (7526). Or check your local white pages under Planned Parenthood.

➤ Your local Planned Parenthood also advocates for reproductive rights in your community and state. There are many ways you can get involved—just look in your local telephone directory and give them a call.

Here are some other sites that offer efficient ways for you to get involved with the reproductive rights movement:

➤ National Abortion and Reproductive Rights Action League (NARAL) has campus organizations and offers an on-line forum for students at **www.naral.org**.

➤ The Feminist Majority Foundation sponsors Leadership Alliances on college campuses with its Choices campaign. Reach them at **www.feministcampus.org**. They also list feminist organizations at **www.feminist.org/gateway/master.html**. Say it loud and proud, please.

➤ Medical Students for Choice is at **www.ms4c.org**.

➤ An education project tailored specifically for young people is the Pro-Choice Public Education Project at **www.protectchoice.org**.

➤ The American Civil Liberties Union is actively involved in fighting parental notification laws, **www.aclu.org**.

➤ For good information and support try Catholics for a Free Choice, **www.cath4choice.org**.

➤ The Religious Coalition for Reproductive Choice, **www.rcrc.org**, sponsors the Spiritual Young for Reproductive Freedom at **www.syrf.org**.

➤ **www.thirdwavefoundation.org** provides organizing tools for young
activists.

➤ **www.choiceusa.org** provides information on campus organizations.

Chapter Fifteen

Motherhood in freedom and fatherhood too

 What a gift motherhood has been to me.

—Hollie, age twenty-nine

My father was full of sayings, like, "There's nothing wrong with me a million dollars wouldn't cure." When I first went to work for Planned Parenthood, he predicted I'd always have a job because "even when people go to the moon, they'll still be screwing."

The process of writing this book, reading all the stories and thinking about my own, led me to ask my children what they remembered about our lives as they were growing up. My son, David, said, "I always knew you were different from most other moms. They let life come to them instead of setting their own trail. You have a desire to learn." The strands of my life eventually and happily intertwined with Alex, who shares my passion for this movement so strongly. Together we have a combined family of six children, nine grandchildren, and one great-grandchild.

There have been so many wonderful changes in women's lives in the years I have worked with Planned Parenthood. Many more pregnancies are planned. Many more unintended pregnancies never occur. There's been a dramatic decrease in teen pregnancies. Many more children are born very wanted. More birth control options exist. Maternal and child health have dramatically improved. A whole generation of young women assumes it is their perfect right to get the education and jobs they want, and to have the family size they want when and if they want it. Not that all problems have been solved, not by a long shot. But the social context in which I write *Behind Every Choice Is a Story* is very different than the world in which I grew up and had my children. We speak today, literally, from a different reality.

Birth control became family planning became reproductive and sexual health. It's not just about birth control and abortion any more, but also about desiring parenthood and being able to achieve it in freedom. It's about the fullness of life for ourselves and our daughters and sons, now and into the future. It is still about wanted children, sexual pleasure, healthy mothers, and emancipated women to be sure. But now we begin with affirmation of childbearing choices instead of a focus solely on cessation of childbearing, love instead of fear, hope instead of despair.

I can see Margaret Sanger smiling in that kaleidoscopic mirror when I think of the many planned families around me, the many happy stories that I am privileged to hear.

But in my own life, what's happened is nothing short of a miracle or, perhaps, a redemption. My children, who thrived in spite of parents who were children themselves, who endured my bumbling efforts not to make the mistakes I felt my parents had made (thereby inventing a whole new set of mistakes), who through no fault of their own had their lives disrupted while I found mine, have experienced the incomparable joy of planned, wanted children. I've had the double bonus of experiencing how the children I gained from my marriage to Alex have also been able to make the choices that were best for them, supported by family and friends and technology, comfortable in a world where planning to have children—or not—is truly a choice. Those who have given birth are incredibly wonderful, nurturing parents. Those who have not are incredibly wonderful, nurturing aunts.

In the short space of a generation, I have had the great privilege of helping change the world, at least for them. I can think of no greater joy.

Have you ever walked among the headstones in an old cemetery? Not only is it filled with the graves of women who died by the time they were forty, exhausted from endless childbearing, but also with the tiny headstones of the many babies who didn't survive. No more. Nor must it be, ever again. That is the mantle all of us who value freedom and justice must wear. We must be eternally vigilant, and we must continue to advance our laws and practices toward greater freedom and justice.

Advanced technology has propelled the changes that have taken place, of course, but it's much more than that. It's a cultural and attitudinal change that is beginning to give women an equal seat at life's table and to honor our unique status as humans who can envision and plan for the future—as co-creators of a better world. Who says dreams don't come true?

The day that my son, David, and his wife, Sally, had their first child, I had proof positive that we do, indeed, live in that world. David told me with tears in his eyes, "Mom, the doctor said that Michael is such a lucky baby to have been born to such good parents." David also said to me that he wasn't a trailblazer like I was, that he wasn't out to change the world, just to raise good kids.

And I thought: David, in the end, that's exactly how we do change the world. One story at a time.

Tell me your story

The earliest humans understood the power of stories. Stories connect us with our fellow humans. They teach and inspire. And they move us to make a better world.

I encourage you to tell your stories. Telling my story in this book helped open up conversations with my children that deepened our relationships. It can do the same for you.

That's the personal part. There's also the political. For too long, reproductive health, sex, and sexuality have been taboo subjects. But the more we tell the personal stories that illuminate these social issues, the closer we will be to creating a society that respects our reproductive rights.

Just as the stories in Margaret Sanger's *Motherhood in Bondage* helped advance the cause of birth control in 1928, so the brave individuals who shared their life-affirming stories in *Behind Every Choice Is a Story* are advancing reproductive rights today.

Telling our stories challenges the disconnect between our real lives and the restrictions set by our institutions. It's easy for Congress or clergy to lay down the law on reproductive rights. But when you hear the story of a woman whose life was saved by access to reproductive health services, dogma and debate go out the window.

Here are three ways you can join the storytelling movement to advance reproductive freedom:

1. Go to **www.behindeverychoice.com**. You'll find an easy format for sharing your story—confidentially if you wish. You can also visit **www.plannedparenthood.org**.

2. Through either Web site, you can get the *Behind Every Choice Is a Story*℠ tool kit. It tells you how to build community through storytelling. It can also help you set the agenda for meetings, and plan teach-ins, speak-outs, speeches, or intimate storytelling salons.

    A special guide will show you how to form your own *Behind Every Choice Is a Story* book club. Learn how to get your story in the newspaper, on the radio, or into the story line for a television show. Find out how it can influence public policy.

    If you're not a writer, don't worry. The power is in your story. Since your story may be used in future books, you will become part of the long history of reproductive choice. Tell your story, change the world.

3. Share stories with your friend, daughter, sister, or parent.

Behind every choice is a story. I want to hear yours.

Bibliography

Bibliography is divided into sections by chapter.

Introduction

Garrow, David J. *Liberty and Sexuality: The Right to Privacy and the Making of Roe v.* Wade. Berkley, California: University of California Press, 1998.

The National Abortion and Reproductive Rights Action League (NARAL) 2002. *Federal and State Legislation: Reproductive Choice Issues.* http://www.naral.org/issues/issues_legislation.html

Planned Parenthood Federation of America, Inc. *Creating Hope for Humanity: Planned Parenthood—Our Story and Vision for the Future,* 2002.

Planned Parenthood Federation of America, Inc. 2002. *Fact Sheet: Planned Parenthood Services 2000.* http://www.plannedparenthood.org/library/BIRTHCONTROL/ Services.html

Planned Parenthood Federation of America, Inc. *Save Roe!* http://www.saveroe.com, 2002.

Sanger, Margaret. *Motherhood in Bondage.* Elmsford, New York: Maxwell Reprint Company, 1928.

Chapter One

The Alan Guttmacher Institute (AGI). *Teenage Sexual and Reproductive Behavior in Developed Countries: Can More Progress Be Made?* http://www.agi-usa.org/pubs/euroteen_or.html, 2001.

Centers for Disease Control and Prevention. Adolescent Health: State of the Nation—Pregnancy, Sexually Transmitted Diseases, and Related Risk Behaviors Among U.S. Adolescents. http://www.cdc.gov/nccdphp/dash/ahson/ahson.htm, 2001.

Darroch, Jacqueline E., D. J. Landry, and Susheela Singh. "Changing Emphases in Sexuality Education in U.S. Public Secondary Schools, 1988–1999." *Family Planning Perspectives* 32: 204–12.

Hoff, Tina and Liberty Greene. *Sex Education in America: A Series of National Surveys of Students, Parents, Teachers, and Principals.* Menlo Park, California: The Henry J. Kaiser Family Foundation, 2000.

The Henry J. Kaiser Family Foundation. *Fact Sheet: Teen Sexual Activity.* 2000. http://www.kff.org/content/2000/3040/TeenSexualActivity.PDF

McGuire, David. *Too Hot to Handle.* Salon.com. http://dir.salon.com/sex/feature/2001/02/05/fox/index.html, 2001.

National Guidelines Task Force. *Guidelines for Comprehensive Sexuality Education,* 2nd ed. New York: Sexuality Information and Education Council of the U.S., 1996.

National Coalition Against Censorship (NCAC). *Abstinence-Only Education: Why First Amendment Supporters Should Oppose It.* http://www.ncac.org/issues/abonlypresskit.html#background, 2001.

Planned Parenthood Federation of America, Inc. *White Paper Adolescent Sexuality.* http://www.plannedparenthood.org/library/sexuality/AdolescSexual.html, 2001.

Satcher, David. *The Surgeon General's Call to Action to Promote Sexual Health and Responsible Sexual Behavior.* Rockville, Maryland: Office of the Surgeon General, 2000.

Schemo, Diana Jean. "Sex Education with Just One Lesson." *The New York Times,* 28 December. A1., 2000.

Siegel, David M.; M.J. Aten and M. Enaharo. "Long-Term Effects of a Middle School- and High School-Based Human Immunodeficiency Virus Sexual Risk Prevention Intervention." *Archives of Pediatric and Adolescent Medicine* 155: 1117-26, 2001.

Chapter Two

The Alan Guttmacher Institute (AGI). *Facts in Brief: Teen Sex and Pregnancy.*
http://www.agi-usa.org/pubs/fb_teen_sex.html, 1999.

The Alan Guttmacher Institute (AGI). *Facts in Brief: Teenage Sexual and Reproductive Behavior in Developed Countries,* 2001

The Alan Guttmacher Institute (AGI). *Facts in Brief: Teenagers' Sexual and Reproductive Health. http://www.agi-usa.org/pubs/fb_teens.html,* 2002.

Fine, Michelle. "Sexuality, Schooling, and Adolescent Females: The Missing Discourse of Desire." *Harvard Educational Review* 58: 29–50. 1988.

Gilligan, Carol. *In a Different Voice.* Cambridge, Massachusetts: Harvard University Press, 1993.

Planned Parenthood Federation of America, Inc. *teenwire.* http://www.teenwire.com, 2002.

Laumann, E.O., J.H. Gagnon, R.T. Michael, and S. Michaels. *The Social Organization of Sexuality: Sexual Practices in the United States.* Chicago: University of Chicago Press, 1994.

Reiss, Ira L. and Harriet M. Reiss. *An End to Shame: Shaping Our Next Sexual Revolution.* Buffalo, New York: Prometheus Books, 1990.

Rickert, Vaughn I., Rupal Sanghvi and Constance M. Wiemann. "Is Lack of Sexual Assertiveness Among Adolescent and Young Adult Women a Cause for   Concern?" *Perspectives on Sexual and Reproductive Health* 34: 178–83, 2002.

Chapter Three

Abma, Joyce, Anne Driscol, and Kristin Moore. "Young Women's Degree of Control   over First Intercourse: An Exploratory Analysis." *Family Planning Perspectives* 30: 12–18, 1998.

Estes, Richard, and Neil A. Weiner. *The Commercial Sexual Exploitation of Children in the U.S., Canada and Mexico.* University of Pennsylvania School of Social Work. http://caster.ssw.upenn.edu/~restes/CSEC_Files/ Complete_CSEC_020220.pdf, 2001.

Hillis, Susan D., Robert F. Anda, Vincent J. Felitti and Polly A. Marchbanks. "Adverse Childhood Experiences and Sexual Risk Behaviors in Women: A Retrospective Cohort Study." *Family Planning Perspectives* 33: 206–211, 2001.

Reiss, Ira L. and Harriet M. Reiss. *An End to Shame: Shaping Our Next Sexual Revolution.* Buffalo, New York: Prometheus Books, 1990.

Chapter Four

American Civil Liberties Union. 2001. *Parental Involvement Laws.* ACLU Reproductive Freedom Project.
http://www.aclu.org/library/parent.html, 2001.

American Academy of Pediatrics. "The Adolescent's Right to Confidential Care When Considering Abortion. " *Pediatrics* 97: 746–51, 1996.

Bellotti v. Baird (Bellotti I), 428 U.S. 132, 1976.

Bellotti v. Baird (Bellotti II), 443 U.S. 622, 1979.

Boonstra, Heather and Elizabeth Nash. "Minors and the Right to Consent to Health Care." *The Guttmacher Report on Public Policy* 3: 4–8, 2000.

Blum, Robert W., Michael D. Resnick and Trisha Stark. "Factors Associated with the Use of Court Bypass by Minors to Obtain Abortions." *Family Planning Perspectives* 22: 158–60, 1990.

Henshaw, Stanley K. and Kathryn Kost. "Parental Involvement in Minor's Abortion Decisions." Family Planning Perspectives 24: 196–207, 1992.

Melton, Gary B. and Nancy Felipe Russo. "Adolescent Abortion: Psychological Perspectives on Public Policy." *The American Psychologist* 42: 69–72, 1987.

The National Abortion and Reproductive Rights Action League (NARAL). *Federal and State Legislation: Reproductive Choice Issues.*
http://www.naral.org/issues/issues_legislation.html, 2002.

Patterson, Richard North. Speech given at "Power of Choice Luncheon." 2 March. National Abortion and Reproductive Rights Action League (NARAL).
http://www.naral.org/mediaresources/press/2001/
pr030201_patterson.html, 2001.

Planned Parenthood Federation of America, Inc. *Fact Sheet: Laws Requiring Parental Consent or Notification for Minors' Abortions.*
http://www.plannedparenthood.org/LIBRARY/ABORTION/
StateLaws.html, 2002.

Planned Parenthood Federation of America, Inc. *Fact Sheet: Teenagers, Abortion, and Government Intrusion Laws.*
http://www.plannedparenthood.org/library/ABORTION/laws.html, 1999.

Planned Parenthood Federation of America, Inc. *Fact Sheet Teenagers, Abortion, and Government Intrusion Laws.*
http://www.plannedparenthood.org/library/ABORTION/laws.html, 1999.

Planned Parenthood v. Casey, 505 U.S. 833, 1992.

Prescott, Heather Munro. *A Doctor of Their Own The History of Adolescent Medicine*. Cambridge, Massachusetts: Harvard University Press, 1998.

Chapter Six

Irish Family Planning Association (IFPA). *Women and Children First— Human Stories.*
http://www.ifpa.ie/campaigns/wcf/stories.html, 2002.

Kaiser Daily Health Policy Report. *Poor Women More Likely to Have Health Problems, Limiting Their Employment Potential, Study Finds.*
http://www.kaisernetwork.org/daily_reports/
print_report.cfm?DR_ID=5872&dr_cat=3, 18 July, 2001.

United Nations Development Fund for Women (UNIFEM). *Eradicating Feminized Poverty.*
http://www.unifem.undp.org/ec_pov.htm, 2002.

United Nations Population Fund (UNFPA). *The Right to Choose: Reproductive Rights and Reproductive Health.*
http://www.unfpa.org/swp/1997/swpmain.htm, 1997.

The United States Agency for International Development (USAID). *Unmet Need for Family Planning.*
http://www.usaid.gov/pop_health/pop/publications/docs/
unmetneed.pdf, 1999.

Burrelle's Information Services, CBS News Transcripts. "Overpopulation in Mexico's Cities Causes Problems," *60 Minutes,* 1991.

Chapter Seven

The Alan Guttmacher Institute (AGI). *Facts in Brief: Induced Abortion.*
http://www.agi-usa.org/pubs/fb_induced_abortion.html, 2000.

Allyn, David. *Make Love, Not War: The Sexual Revolution, an Unfettered History.* Boston: Little, Brown and Company, 2000.

Asbell, Bernard. *The Pill The Biography of a Drug That Changed the World.* New York: Random House, 1995.

Centers for Disease Control and Prevention. *Ten Great Public Health Achievements in the 20th Century.*
http://www.agi-usa.org/pubs/fb_induced_abortion.html, 2001.

Coontz, Stephanie. *The Way We Never Were: American Families and the Nostalgia Trap.* New York: Basic Books, 1992.

Djerassi, Carl. *This Man's Pill: Reflections on the 50th Birthday of the Pill.*

New York: Oxford University Press, 2001.

Donohue, John J. III, and Steven D. Levitt. *The Impact of Legalized Abortion on Crime*. Social Science Research Network Electronic Library. http://papers.ssrn.com/sol3/papers.cfm?abstract_id=174508, 2000.

King, Martin Luther Jr. *Family Planning—A Special and Urgent Concern,* Speech given upon accepting The Planned Parenthood Federation of America Margaret Sanger Award, 5 May,1966.

Montagu, Ashley. *Sex, Man and Society.* New York: G.P. Putnam's Sons, 1969.

NOVA. *18 Ways to Make a Baby.* Broadcast transcript. PBS. http://www.pbs.org/wgbh/nova/transcripts/2811baby.html, 9 Ocotber, 2001.

Skuy, Percy. *Tales of Contraception.* Toronto: History of Contraception Museum, 1995.

Tone. Andrea. *Devices and Desires: A History of Contraceptives in America.* New York: Hill and Wang, 2001.

Chapter Eight

National Committee for Adoption. *Adoption Factbook: U.S. Data Issues, Regulations, and Resources.* Washington D.C.: National Committee for Adoption, 1989.

Solinger, Rickie. *Beggars and Choosers: How the Politics of Choice Shapes Adoption, Abortion, and Welfare in the United States.* New York: Hill and Wang, 2001.

Western Behavioral Sciences Institute, Abortion Policy Task Force. *How To Talk About Abortion*, 1991.

Chapter Nine

The Alan Guttmacher Institute (AGI). State Policies in Brief: Insurance Coverage of Contraceptives. http://www.agi-usa.org/pubs/spib_ICC.pdf, 2002.

Erickson v. Bartell Drug Company 141 F. Supp. 2d 1266 (W.D. Washington, 2001.

Wilson, Alysa, Karen Flyer and Corinne McSpedon. "The Evolution of Women's Health Resources." *The Journal of Gender-Specific Medicine* 2: 54–62, 1998.

Kaeser, Lisa. "What Methods Should Be Included in a Contraceptive Coverage Insurance Mandate?" *The Guttmacher Report on Public Policy,* 1: 1-2, 1998.

The Henry J. Kaiser Family Foundation. *An "Epic" Debate: The Equity in Prescription Insurance and Contraceptive Coverage Act— Contraception Among Privately Insured Women.* http://www.kff.org/content/archive/1408/insured.html, 1998.

Planned Parenthood Federation of America, Inc. *Fact Sheet: Equity in Prescription Insurance and Contraceptive Coverage.* http://www.plannedparenthood.org/library/BIRTHCONTROL/ EPICC_facts.html, 2000.

The U.S. Equal Employment Opportunity Commission. *Decision on Coverage of Contraception.* 14 December. http://www.eeoc.gov/docs/decision-contraception.html, 2000.

Chapter Ten

American Life League. Birth Control—RU-486. http://www.all.org/ issues/nf04.htm, 1996.

Campbell, Catherine. "Mergers Mean Less Access to Abortion Services." *Pro-Choice Action Network.* http://www.prochoiceactionnetwork-canada.org, 2002.

Catholics for a Free Choice. *Hospital Mergers in the USA.* http://www.cath4choice.org/nobandwidth/English/ healthmergers.htm, 2001.

Ellertson, Charlotte, James Trussell, Felicia H. Stewart and Beverly Winikoff. Should Oral Contraceptives Be Available Without Prescription? *American Journal of Public Health* 8: 1092–4, 1993.

Jacoby, Susan. "Under the Knife and the Cross—A Wave of Catholic Hospital Mergers is Curtailing Medical Services, Especially for Women." http://www.tompaine.com/feature.cfm?ID=4382, 2001.

MergerWatch. *Abortions Allowed (again) at South Miami Hospital.* http://www.mergerwatch.org/hospitals/Miami.html, 1998.

O'Donnell, Jayne. Catholic Hospital Deals Limit Access, Activists Say. *USA Today,* 8 April. 1B, 1999.

Planned Parenthood Global Partners. *Why should the United States Support Family Planning Programs in Other Countries?* http://www.plannedparenthood.org/global/matters/index.asp, 2002.

Planned Parenthood Federation of America, Inc. *Fact Sheet: Profiles of 14 Leading Anti-Choice Organizations.* http://www.plannedparenthood.org/library/facts/14anti- choiceFS.html, 2001.

Platt, Leah. "Making Choice Real." *The American Prospect Online.*
    http://www.prospect.org/print/V12/17/platt-l.html, 2001.
Population Action International. *Fact Sheet: How Family Planning Protects
    the Health of Women and Children.*
    http://www.populationaction.org/resources/factsheets/
    factsheet_2.htm, 2002.
Rayman-Read, Alyssa R. 2001. *The Sound of Silence.* The American Prospect
    Online.
    http://www.prospect.org/print/V12/17/rayman-read-a.html, 2001.
Ulmann, Andre. The Development of Mifepristone: A Pharmaceutical
    Drama in Three Acts. *Journal of the American Women's Medical
    Association* Supplement, 3: 117–20, 2000.

Chapter Eleven

U.S. House of Representatives, 107th Congress. Joint Hearing with the
    U.S. Senate Committee on the Judiciary regarding "Partial-Birth
    Abortion: The Truth." *Testimony by Gloria Feldt, Planned Parenthood
    Federation President,*
    http://www.house.gov/judiciary/22234.htm, 11 March,1997.
Bingaman, Jeff and Jon S. Corzine. "Health of the Mother." *The New York
    Times,* 7 February. A29, 2001.
Catholics for a Free Choice. *Actions Speak Louder: Congress Votes on Ameri-
    can Values,* 1993.
Cocco, Marie. "A Long Journey to the Far Reaches of the Far Right."
    Newsday, 14 January. A51, 1999.
Maguire, Daniel C. *Sacred Choices: The Right to Contraception and Abortion
    in Ten World Religions.* Minneapolis, Minnesota: Fortress Press, 2001.
Otto, Mary and Frank Greve. "Barr Denies Urging 2nd Wife into Abortion,
    Criticizes Flynt." *Chicago Tribune,* 13 January. N12. 1999.
Seelye, Katharine Q. Hearing Displays Chasm on Abortion Method. *New
    York Times,* 12 March. A16, 4, 1997.
Schroedel, Jean Reith. Is the Fetus a Person: *A Comparison of Policies Across
    the Fifty States.* Ithaca, New York: Cornell University Press, 2000.
Westchester Coalition for Legal Abortion, Inc. *Pro-Choice Online.*
    http://www.wcla.org/97-summer/su97-04.html, 1997.

Chapter Twelve

Kaiser Daily Health Report. *Reverend Jerry Falwell Says Abortion-Rights Supporters 'Angered God,' 'Helped' Attacks to Happen.* 14 September, 2001.

Roddy, Dennis B. Abortion Stalker Threatens Workers; 'I'm Going to Kill As Many As I Can.' *Pittsburgh Post-Gazette*, 20 June. B-1, 2001.

Clarkson, Frederick. Anti-Abortion Escapee Joins bin Laden on FBI List. *Women's e-news.* http://www.womensenews.org/article.cfm/dyn/aid/668/context/archive, 10 October, 2001.

Clines, Francis X. Man is Arrested in Threats to Abortion Clinics. *New York Times*, 6 December. A20, 5, 2001.

Wolfe, Alan. One Nation After All: What Middle-Class Americans Really Think About God, Country, Family, Racism, Welfare, Immigration, Homosexuality, Work, the Right, the Left, and Each Other. New York: Viking Press, 1998.

Chapter Thirteen

Chesler, Ellen. *Woman of Valor: Margaret Sanger and the Birth Control Movement in America.* New York: Simon & Schuster, 1992.

Lake Snell Perry & Associates/American Viewpoint. *Planned Parenthood Federation of America: A Presentation of Findings Based on a National Survey of 1375 Registered Voters and Four Focus Groups,* 2002.

Melich, Tanya. *The Republican War Against Women.* New York: Bantam, 1996.

Planned Parenthood Federation of America, Inc. *Fact Sheet: A History of Protecting Reproductive Health Rights in the Courts.* http://www.plannedparenthood.org/library/ABORTION/History.html, 2002.

Planned Parenthood Federation of America, Inc. *Report: Major U.S. Supreme Court Rulings on Reproductive Health and Rights (1965–2000).* http://www.plannedparenthood.org/library/ABORTION/majorus.html, 2000.

Planned Parenthood Federation of America, Inc. *Fact Sheet:* Griswold v. Connecticut—*The Impact of Legal Birth Control and the Challenges that Remain.* http://www.plannedparenthood.org/library/facts/griswolddone.html, 2000.

Planned Parenthood Federation of America, Inc. *Fact Sheet:* Roe v. Wade—
    Its History and Impact.
    http://www.plannedparenthood.org/ABORTION/Roe.html, 2002.

Chapter Fourteen

Feldt, Gloria. *Youth Quake The Global Need for Informed Choice.* Planned
    Parenthood Federation of America, Inc.
    http://www.plannedparenthood.org/y6b/YouthQuake.html, 1999.
Optimist International *The Changing Face of the Volunteer: Younger, Busier
    and More Diverse.*
    http://www.optimist.org/archive/mag0101-03.html, 2001.
McManimon, Shannon. *Reflections on 'Resurgent Youth Activism.'* Y&M
    Online.
    http://www.afsc.org/youthmil/html/news/may00/
    youthact%5Fp1.htm, 2000.
Sanger, Margaret. *Margaret Sanger: An Autobiography.* New York: W.W.
    Norton & Company, 1938.

Index